haircults

dylan jones

fifty
years
of
styles
and
cuts

thames and hudson

© 1990 Thames and Hudson Ltd, London
Text © 1990 Dylan Jones

First published in the United States in 1990 by
Thames and Hudson Inc., 500 Fifth Avenue,
New York, New York 10110

Library of Congress Catalog Card Number 89-52218

Printed in Yugoslavia

contents

introduction

the long and short of it

Smart and sassy, sophisticated and sexy, Louise Brooks was one of the cult figures of twenties cinema, star of *Love 'em and Leave 'em*, *Beggars Of Life*, and more. Her short black patent-leather bob was one of the most influential haircuts of the decade, and a style which never seems to date.

'Watch the hair! You know I work on my hair a long time . . . and he hit it. He hits my hair!' So says John Travolta, playing the surrogate medallion man and dancing wizard Tony Manero, in the 1977 smash hit movie *Saturday Night Fever*. After meticulously blow-drying his hair in readiness for a night on the dancefloor at Brooklyn's biggest discothèque, 2001 Odyssey, Travolta – wrapped in a bedsheet to protect his freshly-pressed shirt from his mother's spaghetti sauce – is sitting down to dinner with his family; an argument erupts, and Tony's father swipes him round the head with a fat hand. Outrage; terror; indignation: 'He hit my hair!'

Tony's haircut, lovingly nurtured and regularly trimmed, is the compounded image he projects to the outside world; this is his moniker, his flag, his symbol; you look at Tony Manero's hair and you already know Tony Manero.

A more apparently trifling subject than hair would be hard to find; though it is also unlikely that you could find something, to paraphrase Dick Hebdige, so pregnant with significance. Like the clothes we wear, our haircuts say more about us than we would like to believe. But this is not really a book about haircuts, this is a book about icons and subcultures, about pop stars and film stars, about their journeys to fame and the haircuts they took with them.

This is a catalogue of capillary attraction, of the quiff, the bob, the mohawk, the Beatle cut – a hike through the cultural arteries of the last fifty years, focusing on some of the hairstyles which have become touchstones for their generations – the impressive, the ironic, the iconoclastic, and the just plain

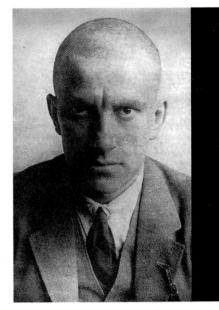

Militant chic: Russian poet Vladimir Mayakovsky combined revolutionary propaganda with efforts to revolutionize poetic technique. He used his haircut to attract attention to his work. This photograph was taken in 1924 by Alexander Rodchenko, the Constructivist designer, with whom he often worked.

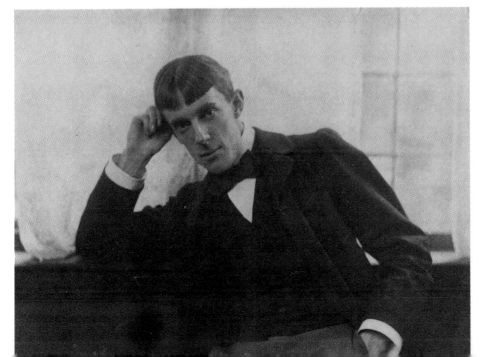

Aubrey Beardsley's style of dress was as flamboyant as his unique Art Nouveau illustrations. And his hair, with its ridiculous centre parting, was a vital ingredient in this 'total look'. It was catalogued for posterity by Frederick Hollyer in 1890, eight years before Beardsley's death.

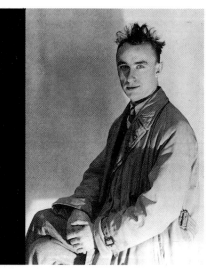

The haircut belonging to French Surrealist Yves Tanguy could easily have turned up in one of his pictures – an amorphous being with no designated form. When he was 36, Man Ray took this definitive photograph of him: a Dadaist portrait of a surreal indulgence. In many ways Tanguy was the first punk.

irritating, from the dandy little forelock which propelled Frank Sinatra to stardom, to the polymorphous perversity of the 1980s, when there was a haircult for everyone.

Throughout the Second World War, American movie stars had a tremendous effect on the way people looked, and not least on the way they wore their hair. Veronica Lake's long blonde peek-a-boo hairstyle became so popular with production line girls that the US Government asked Paramount Pictures to cut it, to avoid any more accidents with machinery. Their hairstyles became so important to these women that many factories built on-site salons in order to curb absences.

And though particular haircuts have always affected the mainstream, it is in the area of youth culture that their significance is most obvious. Ever since Tony Curtis and Elvis Presley tossed their locks in sullen defiance, hair has come to signify rebellion, and the confrontational haircut has been one of the effective tools of teenage insurrection. Every gang since the Mexican Pachucos has been damned by the distinctive tresses of its members – the Teds with their heaving quiffs and dagger combs, the mods with their button-down brush-cuts, the punks with their spiky, heraldic Statues of Liberty, the designer retro-boys with their three-foot hives of mesmeric hair gel... the young generation, the blank generation and the generations with no name have all had haircuts which denote their class, creed and culture. Haircuts have (truly) defined the times in which we live.

before the age of pop

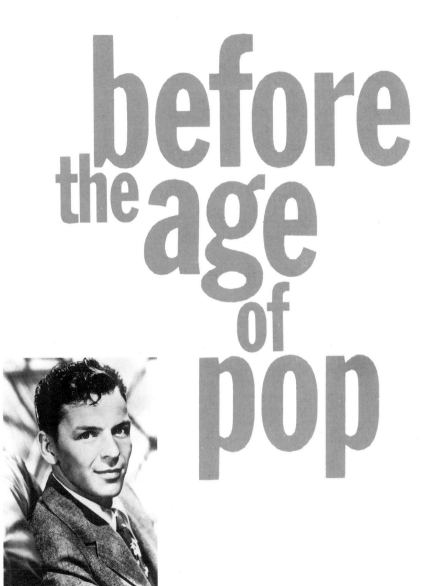

Though teenage rebellion was only just around the bend, during the forties the hairstyles of the young were well and truly rooted in the past. And though the Brylcreem Boys and the Mexican Pachucos were the precursors of the Edwardians and eventually the Teds, it was the film stars and old fashioned crooners who still set the trends. But all that was about to change.

the crew cut

cut across shorty

The American crew cut is living proof that history has a habit of neglecting the truth. This haircut has become synonymous with the All American Boy and his dedication to Uncle Sam, though its origins actually lie in Europe. In the 150 years leading up to the First World War, American Navy regulations governing the haircuts and personal grooming of its personnel were largely concerned with the length and hygiene of beards. During the war, however, the Navy became attracted to the short hair styles adopted by the German forces and American seamen started wearing what has become known as the crew cut.

Initially, hair was only allowed to be one inch long on the top of the head, but by the mid twenties 'this had been increased to two inches. It was changed again in 1948; a memorandum from the Commandant of the

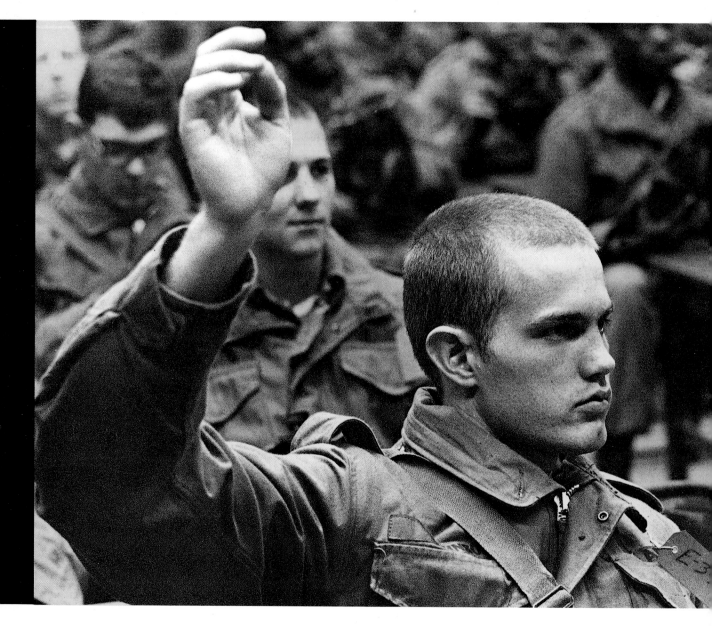

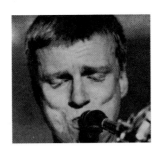

the mulligan

Celebrated baritone saxophonist Gerry Mulligan was admired in the fifties for his innovative pianoless quartet (formed with trumpeter Chet Baker, drummer Chico Hamilton and bassist Carson Smith) but it was his crew cut which brought him notoriety. Mulligan was an exponent of the West Coast school of cool, jazz, lapped up by 'modernist' hipsters in Ray-Bans and turtlenecks.

Mulligan's haircut was definitely 'modernist', positively 'boss', though it happened almost by accident. Tired of consistent disasters with his barbers, who gave him crew cuts which made him look like 'a defrocked monk', he started cutting it himself, combing his hair forward in the process. He is quoted as saying (in *The Hip*, by Roy Carr, Brian Case and Fred Dellar, 1986): 'By the time I was 18 or 19, my hairline was receding. I realized that training my hair back which my mother had done when I was a kid, was breaking the hairs off. I thought, to hell with it, cut all my hair off and brushed it forward. I may have influenced a lot of musicians because I was very much proselytizing the idea that you can save your hair by combing it in its natural direction.'

Marine Corps dated 14 May reads, 'The two inch haircut is an ugly length. (From now on) officers and enlisted men shall, at all times, wear their hair neatly and closely trimmed. The hair may be clipped at the edges of the sides and back, but must be so trimmed as to present an evenly graduated appearance, and must not be over three inches in length. The back of the neck must not be shaved.' Unknowingly, he created a fashion.

The crew cut has enjoyed various periods of popularity with civilians (Steve McQueen and Lee Marvin had two of the more famous crew cuts, as did jazz pianist Bill Evans), declining in recent years in the wake of current distaste for haircuts which don't involve grease. Short hair has always had military connotations, its utilitarian qualities often being exploited by extreme cultural as well as extreme political activists.

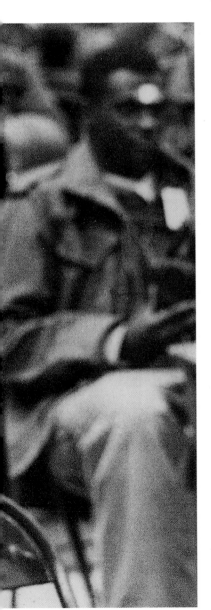

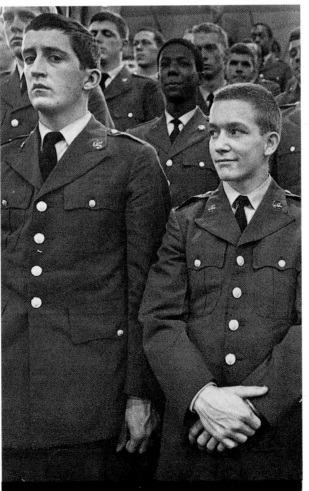

The classic American crew cut: proving that a haircut can be a great leveller.

the argentine duck-tail

Towards the end of the thirties, the working-class Mexican immigrants of the West Coast cities, San Diego and Los Angeles, began to adopt a distinctive style of clothing and haircut. Known as Pachucos, the boys (and sometimes girls) wore dressy zoot suits and duck-tail 'Argentine' haircuts to distinguish themselves from native born North Americans. In 1940 the Pachucos existed pretty much without notice, slowly going about creating their own community; but as soon as America entered the Second World War they began to be discriminated against, not only because of their ethnic origins, but because of their style of dress. In March 1942 the War Production Board created rationing regulations which laid down strict codes concerning the manufacture of suits; zoot suits (because they wasted fabric) were forbidden, and the Pachucos were deprived of their favourite mode of dress in the process. The young Mexicans ignored the rationing, and hundreds of bootleg manufacturers sprang up to cater for the increased demand.

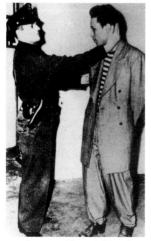

An arresting sight: a Los Angeles police officer pretending to cut the 'Argentine' hairstyle of a young Pachuco, wearing a zoot suit, crew top and a glower.

In June 1943 the tension on the streets of Los Angeles between the armies of recently recruited U.S. servicemen and the zoot-suited Pachucos resulted in a series of infamous riots. This was the duck-tail versus the crew cut, and many Pachucos were beaten up by servicemen, having their suits slashed to shreds and their haircuts scissored off. 'Procedure was standard: grab a zooter. Take off his pants and frock coat and tear them up or burn them. Trim the "Argentine duck-tail" haircut that goes with the screwy costume'. (S. Menelee, *Assignment USA*, 1943).

Towards the end of the war the zoot suit as a fashion hit Britain, but the haircuts remained on the other side of the Atlantic. In terms of American youth culture, the 'Argentine' duck-tail was the first time a haircut had been associated with anything dangerous, and it predates the hairstyles of both the American rockers and the British Teddy boys by at least ten years.

frank sinatra

The Boy from Hoboken

Little Frankie was the sultan of swoon, the original bobby-sox hero, complete with tousled hair and Lincoln cheekbones. The singer was adored by the Sinatratics, the young fans who saw a star in this scrawny little singer with the floppy bowties and the greasy combed-back haircut with the curly forelock. In the early forties Sinatra rapidly became the most popular singer in the world; with his looks and his voice he was made to go to Hollywood.

Swoonatra-mania gradually died, and Frankie tried desperately to reinvent himself, eventually succeeding in 1953 when he took the role of Maggio in Fred Zinnemann's film of James Jones's *From Here To Eternity*. The film won eight Oscars, including Best Supporting Actor for Sinatra. In the fifties the Voice lost his distinctive forelock, and took to wearing hats. His hair, or lack of it, became the bane of his life, and Sinatra was forced to start wearing wigs. In due course he would become as famous for his vast collection of toupees as he had once been for that dandy little forelock.

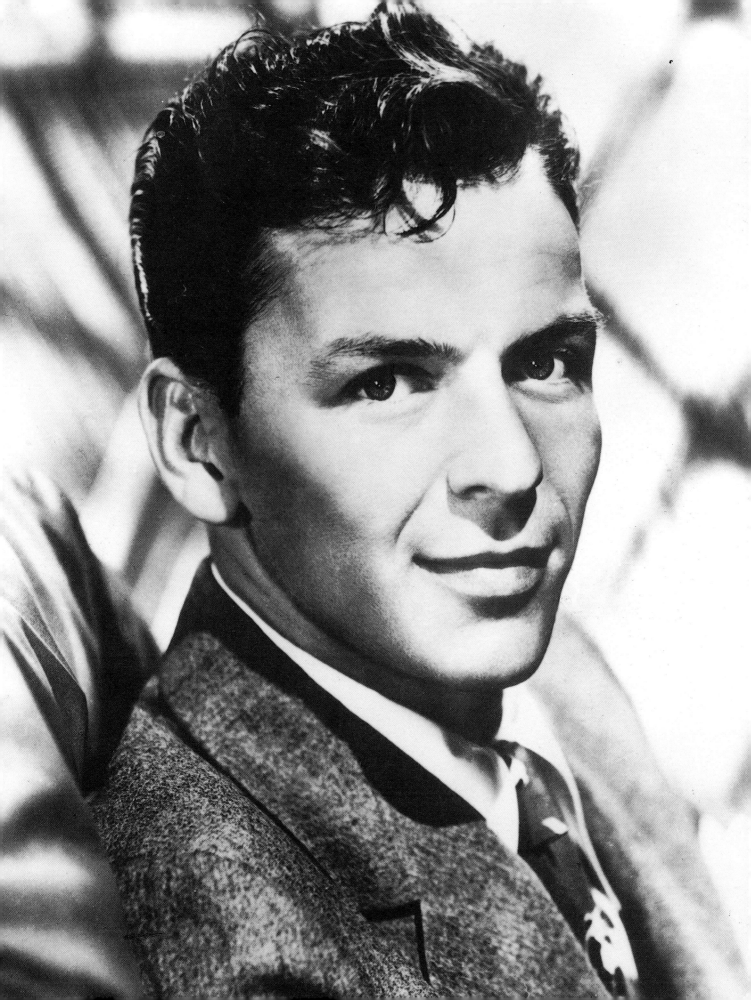

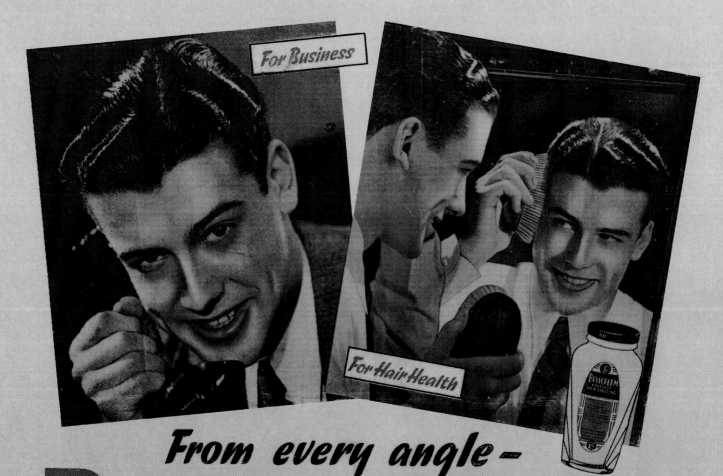
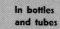

brylcreem boys

When, in 1928, the Birmingham County Chemical Company launched their all-new hair dressing for men, little did they know that their product would eventually help Britain win the Second World War. In 1940 the British Government began issuing 'the smart modern look' to the troops as part of their regulation kit; the Royal Air Force liked the stuff so much that they soon became known as the 'Brylcreem Boys', a tag which remains to this day. This unique hair cream was a hit with civilians as well.

Originally called Elite Hairdressing, Brylcreem was a hybrid of brilliantine and cream. By 1934 it was estimated that some five million British men were Brylcreem users; over a thousand million tubs of the stuff were sold between the fifties and sixties alone. Like Murray's Hair Pomade in the thirties, Brylcreem invited the help of celebrities to sell their product, their most popular campaign involving cricket star Dennis Compton.

The product suffered severe setbacks during the sixties and seventies when wet hair was no longer fashionable but, with the help of an energetic advertising and PR campaign, Brylcreem relaunched itself on the market in the eighties, this time as a trendy accessory for Conspicuous Consumers. The time was right, for there had recently been a boom in the sale of hair gel, water-based haircreams which were being sold as part of the New Lifestyle, in the same way as records, clothes, and style magazines. After revivals of Bass Weejun loafers, Levi 501 jeans, Ray-Ban Wayfarer sunglasses, and countless retro-active consumer durables, why not Brylcreem? The cleverly constructed television ads, posters, style guides and magazine campaigns which followed relaunched the product as a classic of the fifties.

BRYLCREEM GEL

GIVES HAIR THE 'UP-TO-DATE' LOOK

·The easy way to Non Greasy Total Hair Control.

Left: In 1961, in Britain alone, Brylcreem sold over 100 million jars.

The success of Brylcreem's relaunch in the eighties prompted the company to launch Brylcreem Gel, Shampoo, Styling Mousse and various other permutations of the brand.

gentlemen prefer blondes

From 1930 to 1936 Jean Harlow was Hollywood's favourite dime-store blonde (she died in 1937 of uremic poisoning) and her platinum dyed hair was copied across America (she appeared in the film *Platinum Blonde* in 1931). It would be twenty years before Hollywood found a blonde as contentious, or as popular.

Marilyn Monroe was the ultimate sexual grenade, pneumatic and hopelessly flirtatious. Never completely reconciling her publiic and private personas, her sexuality seemingly a burden in both, the world's most recognizable sex symbol was continually trying to rationalize her fame, mostly without success; Monroe was always the lonely beauty.

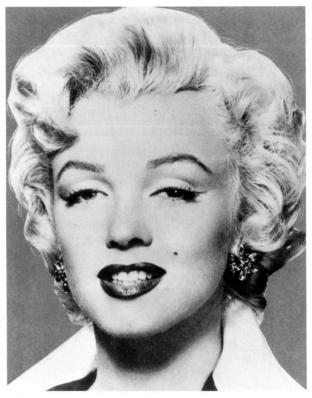

'She played stupid girls who thought they were smart', says Julie Burchill (in *Girls on Film*, Virgin Books, 1986), 'but she was a smart girl who thought she was stupid. She played girls to whom everything came easily . . . but her life seemed to be one constant miscarriage'.

Since her tragic death Monroe has become one of America's most durable twentieth-century icons, along with Mickey Mouse, Coca-Cola and Elvis Presley – her thick blonde curls iconographic proof that, though they might not always have more fun, blondes at least last forever.

The ultimate blonde on film, Marilyn was also granted the status of icon by Andy Warhol in his canvas silkscreen of 1962.

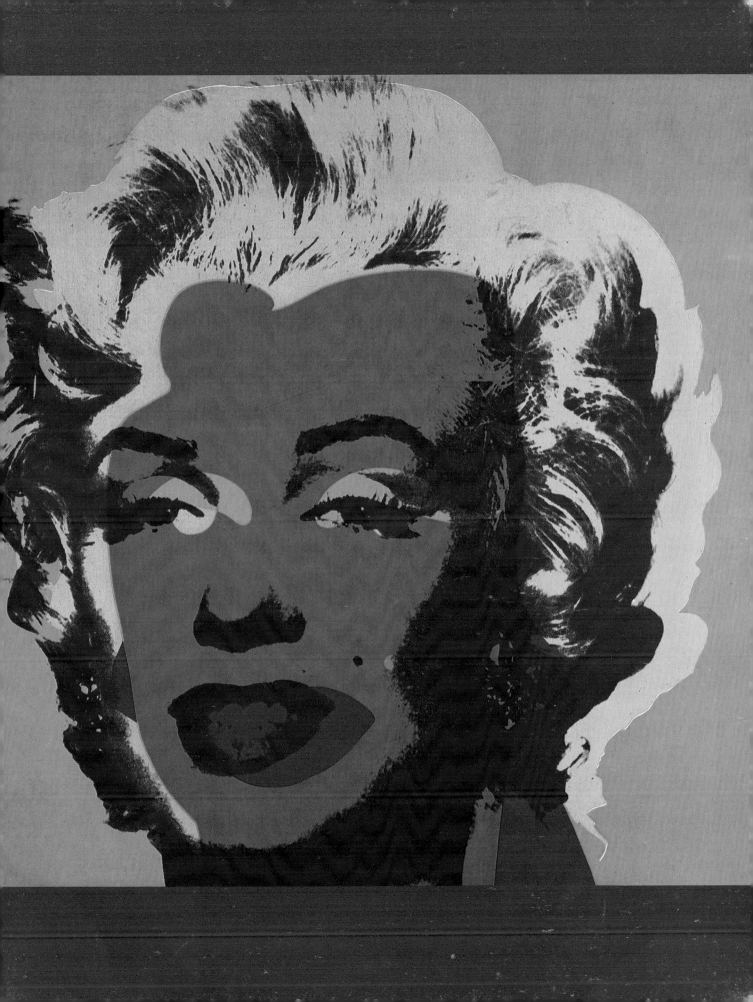

THAT'S THE STYLE

BRYLCREEM

YOUR HAIR

Give your hair the Double Benefit of Brylcreem's Pure Emulsified Oils...

Men who hit the headlines know that smartness counts—and count on Brylcreem for perfect grooming. It works in two ways— (1) Brylcreem grooms without gumming, restoring gloss to the hair. (2) Brylcreem's pure emulsified oils, with massage, have a valuable tonic effect, preventing Dry Hair and Dandruff. Treat your hair handsomely — Brylcreem your hair.

BRYLCREEM—THE PERFECT HAIR DRESSING

dawn of the icon

The fifties saw the haircut really come into its own. Even the haircuts of the late forties tended to have a utilitarian look about them. Then Tony Curtis, James Dean and, most important of all, Elvis Presley brought in the age of the Haircult.

From the opening years of the decade, the youth culture of the western world found itself with a new weapon in its sartorial armoury – a mass of pomaded hair swept back and combed round, the D.A.

——————

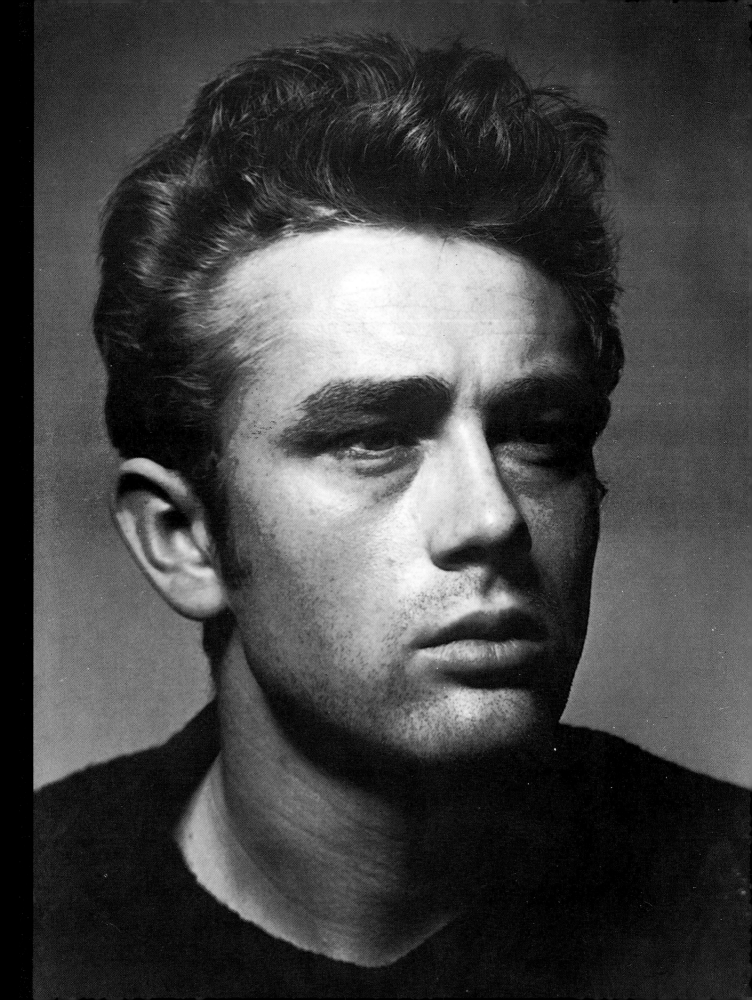

joe cirello and the d.a.

From D.A. to D.O.A.

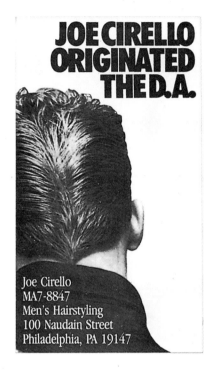

JOE CIRELLO ORIGINATED THE D.A.

Joe Cirello
MA7-8847
Men's Hairstyling
100 Naudain Street
Philadelphia, PA 19147

During the forties, and particularly the fifties, the initials D.A. became associated with the Duck's Ass (instead of District Attorney), a haircut with overlapping wings from the side of the head to the back. This style was popular with British and American youths of the fifties, though the invention of the D.A. is credited a decade earlier to a South Philadelphia barbershop owner called Joe Cirello.

In an interview with Jeffrey Ferry published in *The Face* in 1985 the then seventy-year-old man was quoted as saying, 'I invented the D.A. in 1940 at 6th and Washington Avenue, on a blind kid. I was just playing around, I had something in mind – I figured this kid can't see what I'm doing, so I kept on practising. And then the kids started coming in from Southern High (the neighbourhood school), they said, "Hey, that looks great, try it on me." '

Joe later worked as a staff hairdresser at Warner Brothers Studios in Hollywood, cutting the famous coifs of Frank Sinatra, Wallace Beery, Eddie Fisher, Humphrey Bogart, Bill Haley, Presley himself ('he was crazy, bombed out most of the time'), and even James Dean. 'I was getting ready to go home one day, and he barged in and said, "I got a special engagement tomorrow, I need just a clean-up, clean me up Joe." I cleaned him up. Two days later he was killed in an automobile accident. I was the last person to cut his hair.'

Joe Cirello, creator of the D.A. and the last person to cut Jimmy Dean's hair.

james dean

The cult with a mean mane

James Dean (*opposite*) was, in the words of Dennis Hopper (who starred with the existential idol in *Rebel Without A Cause*), 'the first guerilla artist ever to work in movies.' This hypnotic teen archetype was, *is*, North America's most idolized Neurotic Boy Outsider, the original angst-ridden moody adolescent, whose final car crash placed him forever in celluloid freeze-frame. Though Dean's carefully cultivated persona seemed partly derived from Marlon Brando and Montgomery Clift, his hair was all his own. His biographer David Dalton recalls how the Mutant King created 'a jagged wave', 'the pentecostal flame that became his symbol' from his 'smouldering, unruly bush'. Dean's hair

really was his trademark, a tousled, sullen mass of sexy locks, to which he constantly drew attention by running his hand through them.

Shortly after filming the 'Last Supper' scene in what was to be his last film, *Giant*, on 30 September 1955 at 5.45 pm. Dean crashed his Porsche Spyder 550 into a Ford sedan at the intersection of routes 466 and 41 in California. Ironically, Dean died incomplete; shortly before, his hair had been cut by Joe Cirello, then his famous mane was shaved back from his forehead for the scene, so he died looking thirty years older than he actually was. (Such is the fascination for Jimmy Dean that memorabilia includes bloodstained locks of his hair, retrieved from the wreckage of the crash.) James Dean might not have been the voice of his generation, but he certainly had the mannerisms . . . and the hair.

Left: **The defiant nabob of sob, James Dean had a haircut which cried out for attention.**

tony curtis

The Italian Cut

Tony Curtis spent his whole career trying to live down his haircut. Plucked out of obscurity in 1948 and foisted on to a Hollywood community which didn't take too kindly to upstarts from the Bronx, Curtis had a hard time fitting in. He arrived in Hollywood accompanied by a mane of heavily greased hair curled into a ruffled wedge – a feature the publicity agents at Universal Studios decided to exploit. From thereon Tony Curtis was known as much for his hair as for his acting talents. Critics called him the 'Baron of Beefcake', or 'the boy with a bunch of grapes where his fringe should be'; and generally criticised him for being tremendously good looking. In the end their attentions got to him.

The Tony Curtis haircut (its main features being a curled coif on the forehead, a semi-crew cut top and a full nape) was first acknowledged in his second film, Maxwell Shane's *City Across The River* (1949) and his popularity continued to grow through pictures like *Johnny Stool Pigeon* (1949) and *The Prince Who Was A Thief*

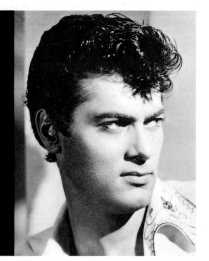

(1951). In nearly every film he made during the fifties he wore this finger-combed ball of grease, even in period pieces like *The Purple Mask* (1955) and Stanley Kubrick's *Spartacus* (1960).

Curtis himself came to detest the attention paid to his looks: 'The Tony Curtis haircut was a phoney. It all began because I couldn't afford a haircut,' he once said. 'Then I thought my very gift was something so mystical and magical that by cutting my hair I thought it would be gone. I could understand what Samson felt. I was afraid if they cut my hair too much they would cut my talent.'

His hair was in fact cut, little locks of it being scissored and sent off to adoring fans by over-eager PR men. The Tony Curtis cut was to influence an entire generation of juvenile delinquents, and give Elvis Presley the model for his own style. This must have seemed ridiculous to little Bernard Schwartz, the Bronx boy who spent the first six years of his life wearing the long plaits which symbolized his Jewish Orthodox roots. 'In the history of things movie-wise I'll probably rate a three line entry as the character who gave a hairstyle to the Teddy boys of the fifties,' he said.

Throughout the fifties the Bronx roughneck wore his heavily greased mop in nearly every movie he made, whether it was appropriate or not.

elvis presley

'Before Elvis there was nothing . . .' (John Lennon)

Although Elvis Presley's haircut is considered to be one of the most influential pop icons of the twentieth century, it was actually copied from Tony Curtis. Presley wore Royal Crown hair pomade during high school to make his blondish locks appear darker. But it wasn't until he saw Tony Curtis in the 1949 movie *City Across The River* that Elvis adopted his greased duck-tail. Of the eleven billed principal actors, Curtis was tenth, but his impact was immeasurable, and his dark greasy hairstyle was copied the world over. So it was that, in the summer of 1951, Elvis finally fashioned his extraordinary hair – a Tony Curtis, dyed blue black, covered in grease with sideburns trailing his cheeks – what *Time* magazine later called 'five inches of buttered yak wool'.

To middle-class white America Elvis Presley was the devil incarnate, a southern white boy who danced and sang like a black. He was threatening because he was so flagrantly *dirty*, owning, among other things, the world's sexiest haircut, a great heavy mop of grease which took his stunning profile way up into the clouds, into dreamland. His truck driver sideburns and curled lip only added to this animal sexuality. In *Elvis World* (1987) Jane and Michael Stern describe the crowning glory: 'Hair is his tradmark and his strength. It has a life of its own, more than the sum of the parts that critics inventory and fans dote over – the sideburns, the wave, the fendors, the duck's ass. Like the man to whose scalp it is attached, the hair breaks loose onstage. Appearing first as a unitary loaf of high-rise melted vinyl etched with grooves along the side, it detonates at the strike of the first chord. It hangs low and dirty, it whips to the beat, it clings like a greedy lover to the sweaty skin on Elvis's neck.' Many people have endured plastic surgery in order to look like Elvis, but none have ever been able to reproduce his hair.

When he appeared for the third time on The Ed Sullivan Show on 6 January 1957, he was shot from the waist up, because his wild erotic dancing had caused an uproar all across America. In reality it made no difference whatsoever, because people could still see his hair.

Elvis kept his mousey hair dyed black all through his career (using everything from Clairol Black Velvet to L'Oréal Excellence Blue Black), originally to carve himself an image, then because he thought it photographed better on film, and finally because he started to go grey (when Elvis died the hair underneath his dye was almost white).

Right: **Elvis was not quite the American original, his haircut having been stolen from Tony Curtis.**

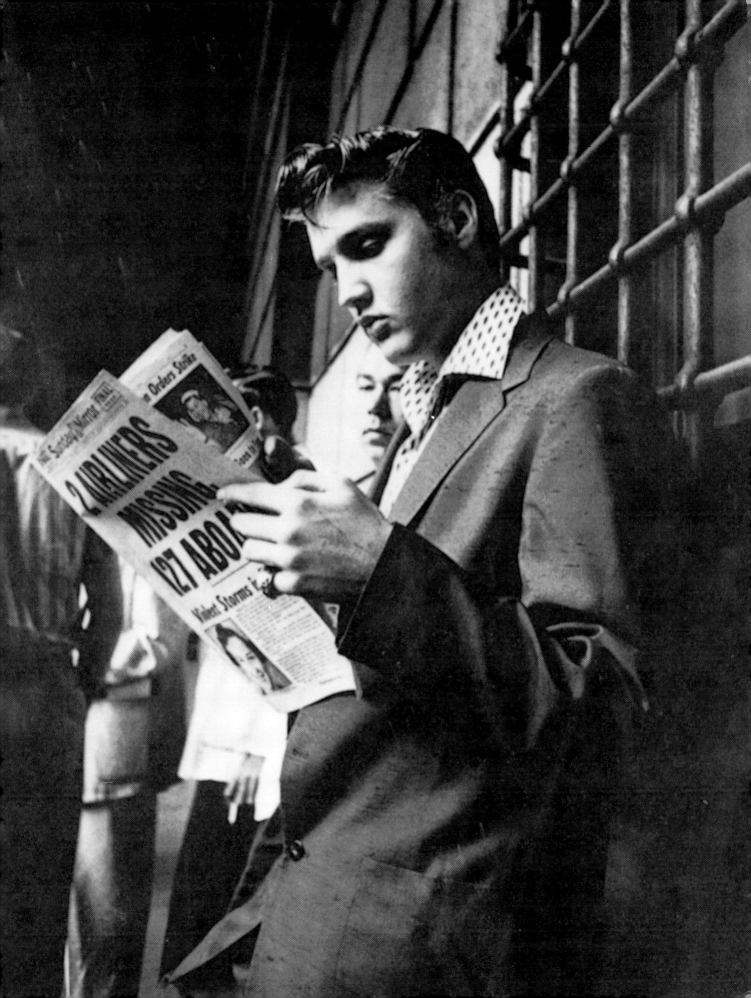

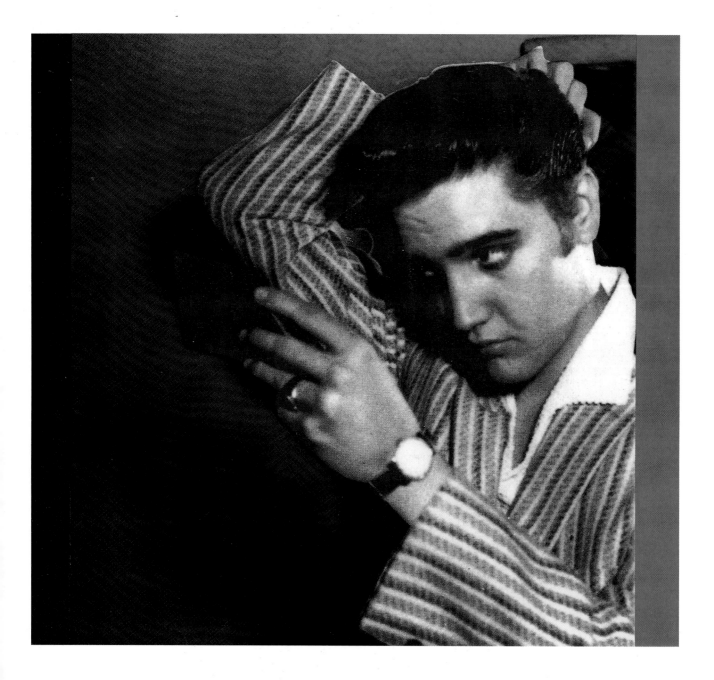

sculpting the quiff

In 1942, the thing which made the majority of American teenage girls go ape was Sinatra bursting into song. In 1956 the sight of Elvis combing his hair provoked the same reaction. Elvis loved to comb his hair, and he was loved for it; it was flagrant narcissism, something which teenage America was just beginning to come to terms with. More than this, Elvis pushing his hand through his hair meant the same as Elvis grabbing his crotch, the same as Elvis stroking his hips or caressing a microphone – it meant sex. His voice was terrific, his dress sense almost futuristic, and he could dance like no other white boy had danced, but the sexiest thing about Elvis Presley was always his hair.

elvis presley

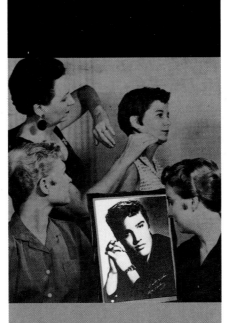

girls on top

During the spring of 1957, *Life* magazine ran a story about a large group of teenage girls from Grand Rapids, Michigan, who were all having their hair cut like Presley. The hairdresser responsible was quoted as saying that she had cut over a thousand 'Elvis heads', and rather optimistically stated that by the following year over 75,000 girls would be wearing it. As this didn't happen, one can only assume that the female portion of teenage America had heard Elvis say that he originally based his huge lacquered conk on the hairstyle worn by some Southern truck drivers.

the end of an era

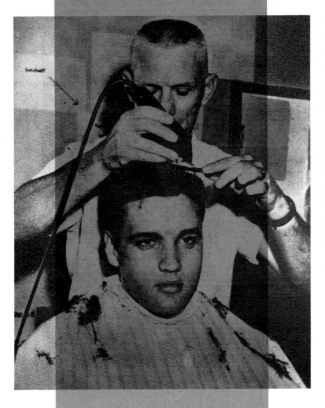

Elvis joined the U.S. Army on 24 March 1958, at the height of his success, becoming serviceman US53310761; twenty-four hours later he lost his famous locks in one of the most photographed events of his career. The photographers begged the barber to cut more slowly, and *Life* magazine collected 1200 pictures from the session. Elvis is reported to have muttered, 'Hair today, gone tomorrow'. The clippings were swept up and destroyed, but the cutting

of the Presley mane had been more symbolic than anyone realized. It not only put a stop to Elvis's brief period of musical creativity, it also signified the end of the first, finest era of rock 'n' roll. When Elvis joined the army it effectively finished his career. His demonic presence was forced to lope about in third-rate beach movies throughout the sixties. The U.S. Army symbolically castrated Elvis, and though he looked pretty similar when he returned two years later in March 1960, things were never the same. As John Lennon said, on being informed of Elvis's death in 1977: 'Elvis died the day he went into the army.'

teds

British Teddy boys caused the first youthquake. The real beginning of post-war youth culture, the Teds were Britain's first teenagers, the first generation to talk with their clothes, their fists and their haircuts. The Teds were not only one of the first truly iconoclastic youth cults, they were also the first group of young people this century to combine aggression with style – they were confrontational for the sake of it. They were the first group of working-class teenagers to express their anger, frustration and youthful energy through their dress. Their neo-Edwardian clothes were a public display of both class and style theft, while their shocking hair was meant as a challenge to the public at large.

Teds took the Edwardian look and mixed it up with elements from the spiv, the Pachuco and the western gunfighter: urban cowboys with creepers, drainpipes, brocade vests, riverboat lace ties, brass rings, velvet half-collared fingertip drapes and daggers. Their stylistic expression of teenage values was the blueprint for every major youth cult which followed. But it wasn't just their clothes, their rituals and their attitude which set them apart from everyone else in 1953 Britain – it was their hair. In his 1971 book *Today There Are No Gentlemen – The Changes in Englishmen's Clothes Since the War*, Nik Cohn wrote: 'Their greatest glory was their sideburns, which had to sprout well past the ear-lobe, and their hair. which was worn long and swept up in a quiff at the front then dragged back at the sides and slopped down heavy with hair oil'. This was the duck's arse, and though the classic tailored D.A. is one of the few hairstyles which has transcended the era in which it was born, the Teds originally wore a variety of different haircuts. The D.A. was also known as the duck-tail; there was also the simple quiff, either combed up, over the forehead or down, in front of it; the elephant trunk, where the duckfins were curled and trained to meet just above the nose; the diamond and silver-dollar crew cuts; the full Tony Curtis; the square-neck Boston; and even the Apache, a variation on the Mohawk. And then later there were the sideburns, inspired by Elvis and often simulated with burnt cork. Grease was important, as it was impossible to keep these creations aloft without some help (or capillary magnetism), though often Teds would use anything available.

Teddy inevitably went mainstream, due in most part to the sudden outbreak of rock'n'roll in 1956; this development was ironic, since the original Teds were not much interested in music; they

**'They bomb styles in clothes, speech and haircuts'
(Emmett Grogan, *Ringolevio*, 1972)**

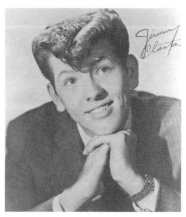

American pin-up Jimmy Clanton in 1958, with a perfect elephant trunk, one of the more eccentric fifties haircuts.

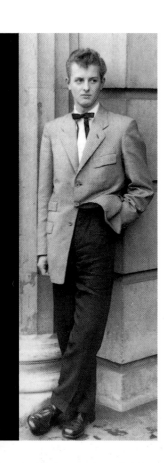

the edwardians

The new Edwardian style was the first British male haircut of the twentieth century to differ radically from the norm; it was also part of Britain's first youth cult. The name 'Edwardians' was originally bestowed upon London Guards officers of the late forties who began dressing in a mock-Edwardian style. The craze was then taken up by the homosexual community and then appropriated by the working classes, who mixed the brocade and velvet extravagances of the Edwardian style with some remnants from the spiv ('suspicious itinerant vagrant') look, to create the New Edwardian look, or what became known as the Ted style.

The New Edwardians wore their hair in the brushed D.A. style, with small quiffs and lots of grease. Teds were on their way.

were, to quote Jon Savage (*i-D* magazine, 1986), bonded by class, clothes and attitude. Perversely, Elvis Presley became the Teds' living god; though they were a very British phenomenon, the Teds' music came almost exclusively from the States. By 1958 in Britain the whole thing had been diluted, though the Ted myth had travelled to Australia (the bodgies, and their female counterparts, widgies) and even Japan (in the form of the Tokyo *tayozoku*).

The Teds, at the height of their early notoriety, are best summed up by Nik Cohn: 'I am different; I am tough; I fuck.'

Seminal duck's arse: Dave Taylor, as illustrated on the cover of his *Jive Jive Jive* LP.

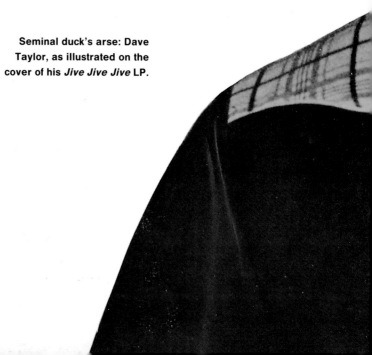

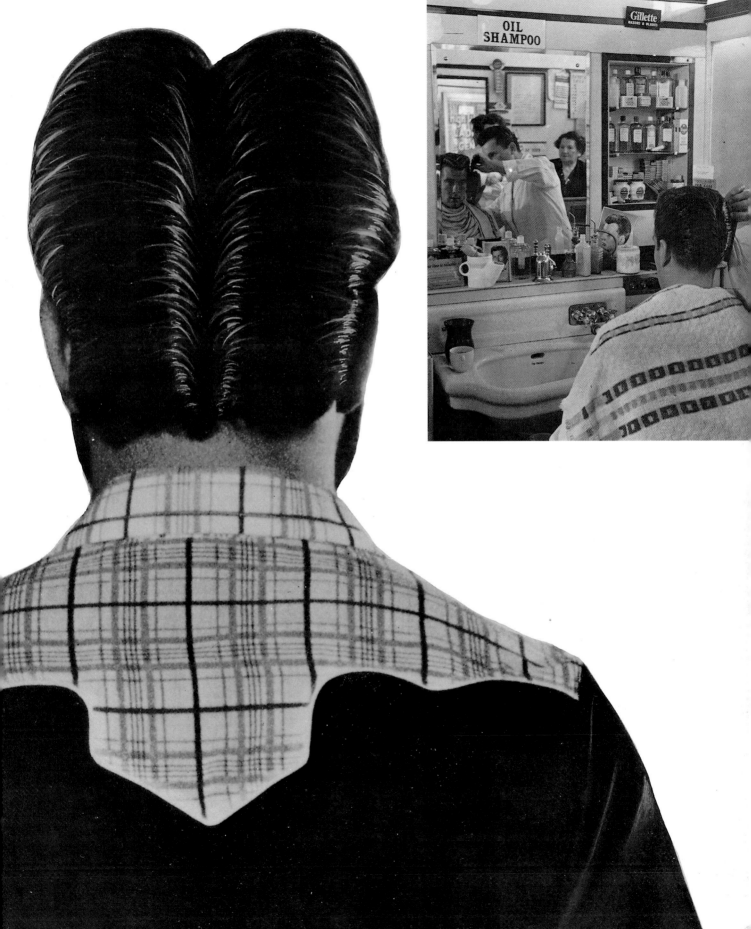

A British Ted getting his
hair cut in 1954.

rockabilly

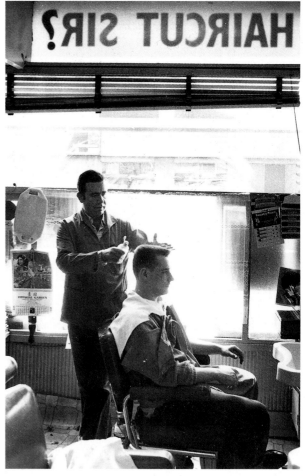

In 1979 in Britain, especially in London, came the rebirth of the rockabilly, a Po-Mo rebel who identified with groups such as the Polecats, the Stray Cats, the Rockats, the Shakin' Pyramids and the Stargazers. During the heady days of punk rock, three years earlier, Teddy boys had been seen as a reactionary breed of old men – dinosaurs still roaming the earth in bright red brothel creepers and luminous socks. The new rockabillies, all between the ages of fifteen and twenty-five, went one step back and three steps forward in terms of style. Not content to dwell in the past, they demanded their own distinctive versions of classic forties/fifties dress, music and haircuts. Rockabilly cuts were enormously popular during the early eighties, and became as much a part of the times as the new romantics, with whom they brushed shoulders and quiffs in clubs from Torbay to Tyneside. Later rockabilly would mutate into psychobilly, neo-hillbilly, quiffabilly and other sub haircults.

mac curtis

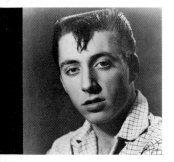

A tonsorial masterpiece, Mac Curtis's haircut is the ultimate rockabilly with a brush flat-top and greased tailfins. Popular in the American South since the late forties (originating from a G.I. cut), it was brought into the public eye in 1956, worn by rockabilly star Mac Curtis. A country singer and radio DJ, in the wake of Elvis, Wesley Ervin Curtis had reinvented himself as a mutant 'billy' (the bizarre mixture of country and hillbilly) on signing with King Records in 1956.

Mac Curtis was nothing if not influential. Towards the end of the fifties the spirit-level comb was introduced to cope with the increased demand for flat-tops by American rockabillies and their highschool clones. Flat-tops started to be worn *en masse* in 1956, but typically the nation's hairdressers were ill-equipped (one Wisconsin barber was reduced to attaching a telescopic arm to his electric clippers, to ensure 'geometric precision'). Approximately thirty per cent of American boys were alleged to have worn flat-tops during this period. The Mac Curtis swept England in 1980 due to the enormous rockabilly revival.

short cuts, london sw2

During the height of the rockabilly revival in 1981, Andy of Andy's Cut'n'Blow Dry in Tulse Hill, Brixton, became the most sought after barber in London. People came from all different part of the capital to have Andy turn their nondescript crops into masterful facsimiles of the Mac Curtis flat-top. But though he specialized in this cut, he actually found it a chore, and was quoted in *The Face* magazine in August 1981 as saying '…it's the German crop with a flat-top, the worst haircut you can get, because it takes so long.'

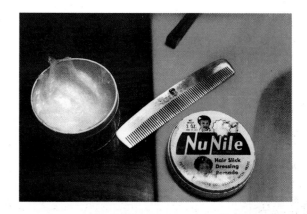

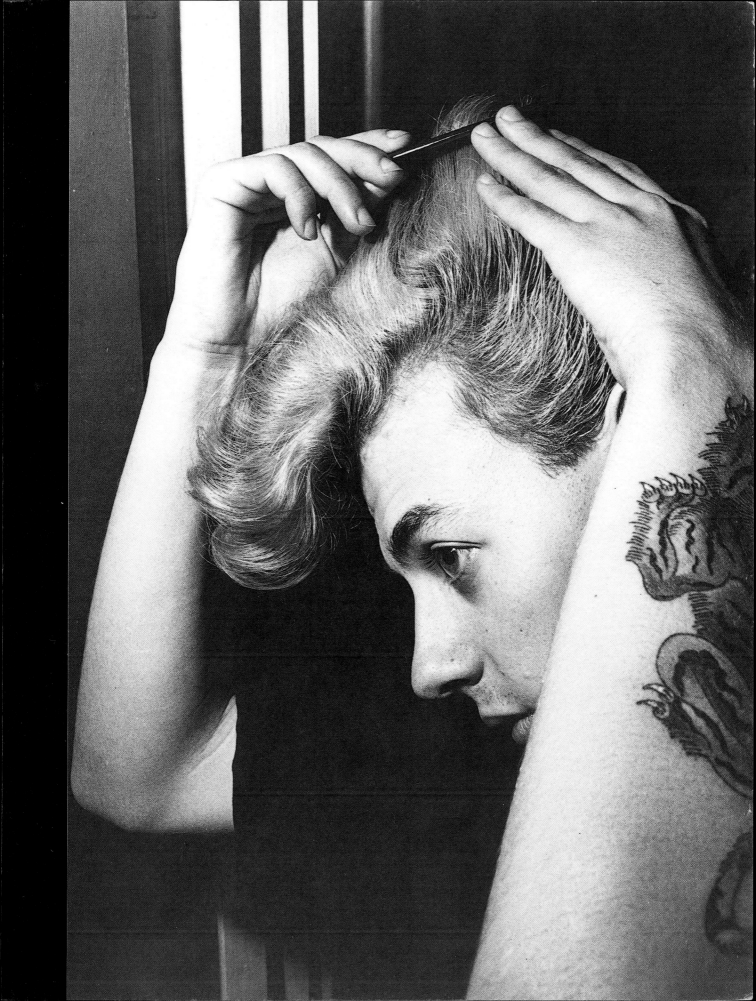

leather boys

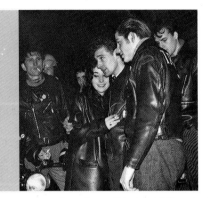

As Teds became sucked into mainstream culture, so the rockers flourished, brandishing their gleaming bikes, their drainpipe trousers, PVC jackets, and long greasy quiffs. Whereas the Teds had copied their style from the Edwardian aristocracy, the rockers borrowed theirs from the hoodlums of American cinema, notably Marlon Brando in *The Wild One* (1953). The film was banned in Britain for fifteen years (eventually surfacing in 1968) but its mystique still travelled, influencing the *blousons noirs* (black jackets) in France and the *skinnknuffe* (leather jackets) in Sweden as well as the rockers in Britain and the folk devils of many other European countries. (Strangely, many rockers never actually saw the film which determined their mode of dress.)

The rockers were the first mobile juvenile delinquents (the American Hell's Angels being considerably older), and consequently their clothes were more functional than those of the Teds. The black leather jacket replaced the drape as the symbol of disgruntled youth, though the rockers' hair was pretty much identical to the Teds, if a little longer. In the early fifties rockers wore their hair in several nondescript styles (they had to wear helmets), but by the beginning of the sixties they all wore their hair like Elvis, in aggressive, greasy quiffs. The rockers spent 1964 on various British beach fronts warring with the mods, gaining themselves a second helping of publicity; but by the end of the decade these parochial cowboys had degenerated into greasers or greboes, the lumpen longhairs of motorcycle culture.

Since the late forties the myth of the motorcycle outlaw has grown to epidemic proportions. British bike boys, or rockers as they became known, greased their hair into long quiffs and dressed in denim jeans. They aspired to leather jackets, though often wore PVC.

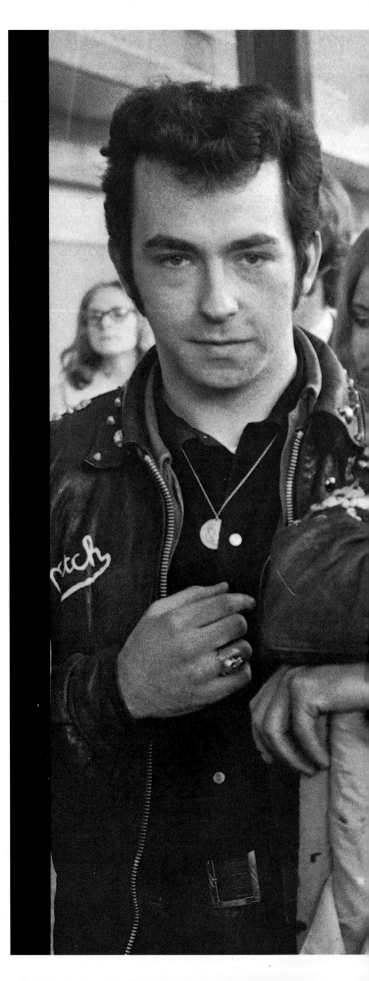

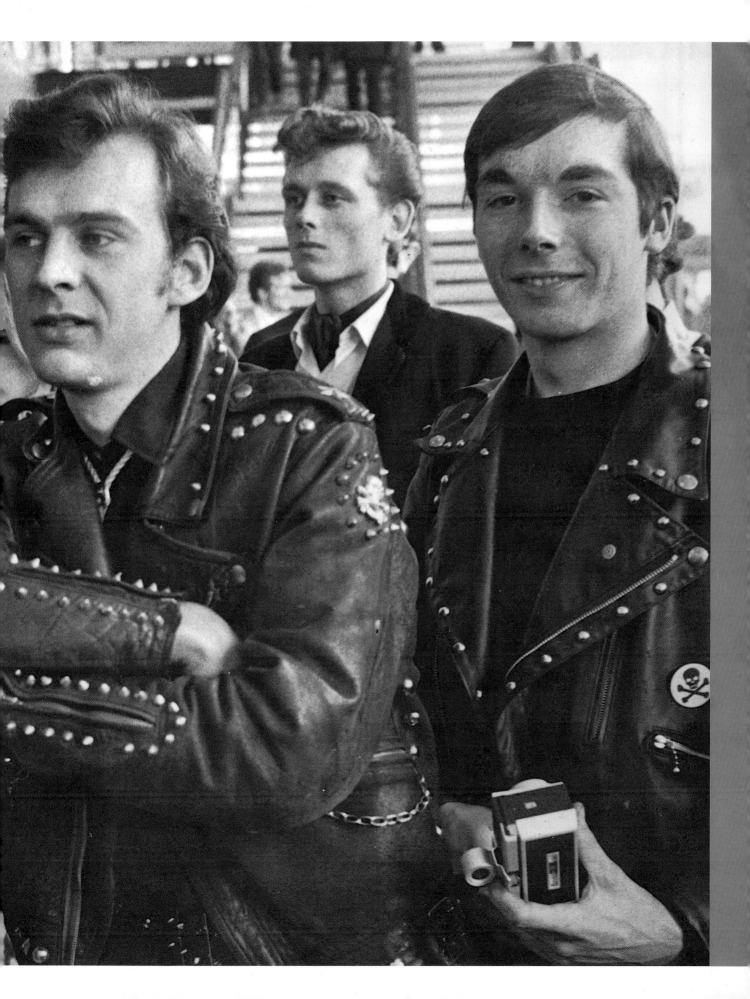

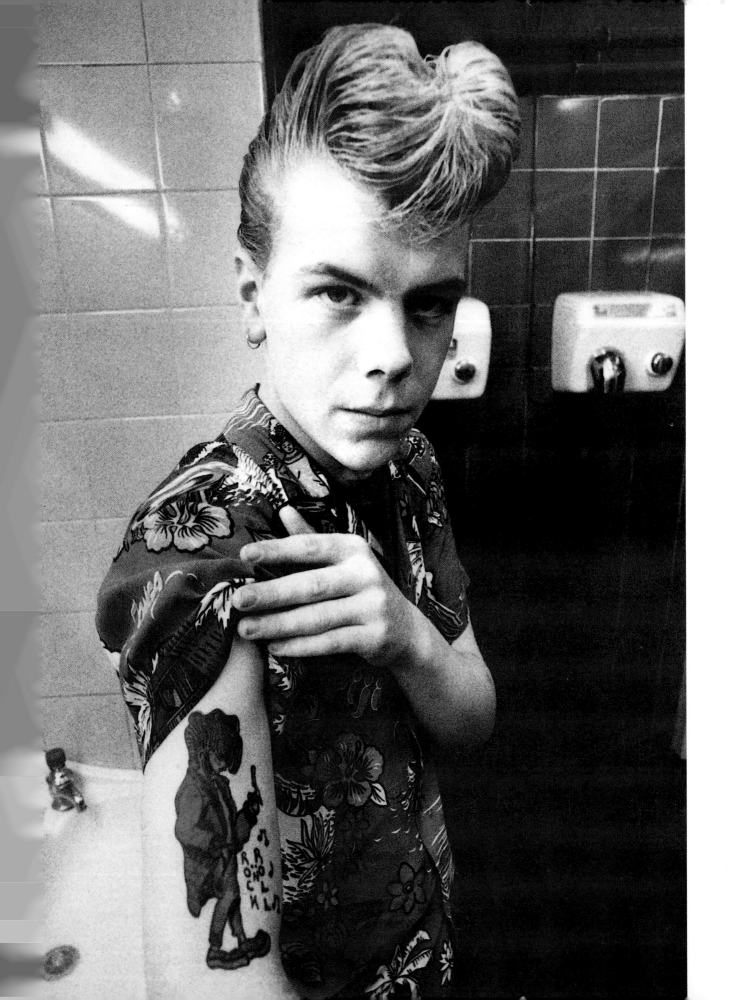

retro-teds

The Teds became London's first urban cowboys, obsessively patrolling their turf whilst stalking other people's. Hair was their most powerful weapon, especially the extraordinary elephant trunk.

In the summer of 1986 photographer Nick Knight was asked by Stephen Bayley, then of The Boilerhouse in the Victoria & Albert Museum, to recreate some of the more influential British youth cults of the last thirty years for an exhibition entitled '14:24 British Youth Culture' which set out to chart the rise of the British teenage consumer since the Second World War. Most recreations of the Teds' mid-fifties uniform tend to be excruciating parodies, usually ham-fisted characterizations by downmarket pop groups or cabaret entertainers. They inevitably focus on the lurid pink drapes and monstrous brothel creepers only worn by holiday camp comics, ignoring the Edwardian finery of their waistcoats, western ties, and lovingly sculpted hair.

There is a common misconception that the British Ted looked like a funfair wideboy, whereas in fact he looked more like a cross between a forties cosh boy and an undertaker, a Byronic gunfighter with thin shoes and wide hair.

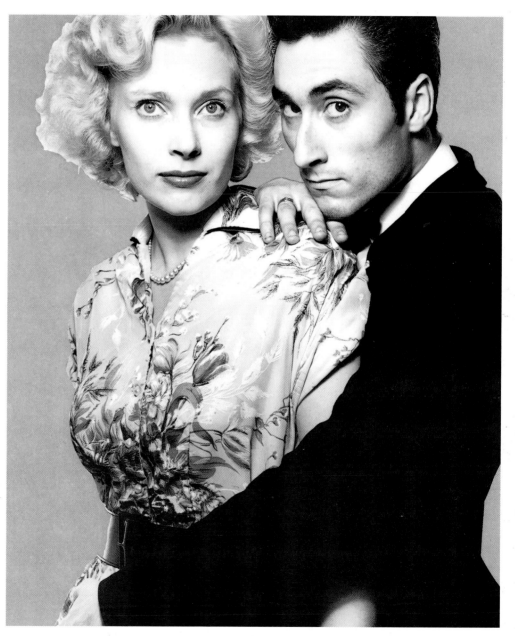

orient boys and stray cat strut

Like many rehabilitated hairstyles, Stray Cat Brian Setzer's 1980 quiff was more extravagant and more expressive than any haircut from the fifties. A towering jumble of long hair, super-gel, retro-dye, and industrial-strength spray, Setzer's D.A. somehow defied gravity.

the wah-ching

According to Tom Wolfe, Hong Kong-born Chinese gang members were the last tee-nagers in America to wear the seminal fifties haircut, the 'teased pompadour with the ducktail'. Over thirty years later the global appropriation of the original youthquake is still going strong. In Yoyogi Park in the Harajuku district of Tokyo, Japanese Teddy boys sport immaculately carved quiffs, 'their sleek Asian hair gelled into tensile apostrophes across their foreheads', as Nicholas Coleridge puts it in *The Fashion Conspiracy* (1987).

Here the young style fanatics promenade in front of each other like some kind of fancy dress parade, with fanatical attention to detail, reproducing the haircuts of long forgotten singers, B-movie actors and hoodlums from the fifties. Soho might produce some specta-cular ducktails, but the parks of midtown Tokyo are where the big quiffs hang out.

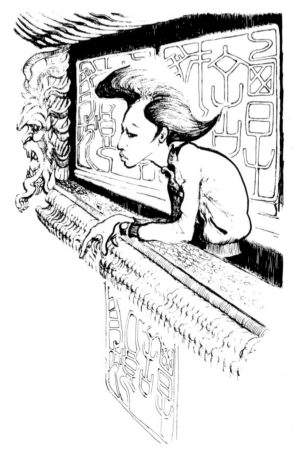

Wah Ching boy, Chinatown, San Francisco, 1969.
Drawing by Tom Wolfe.

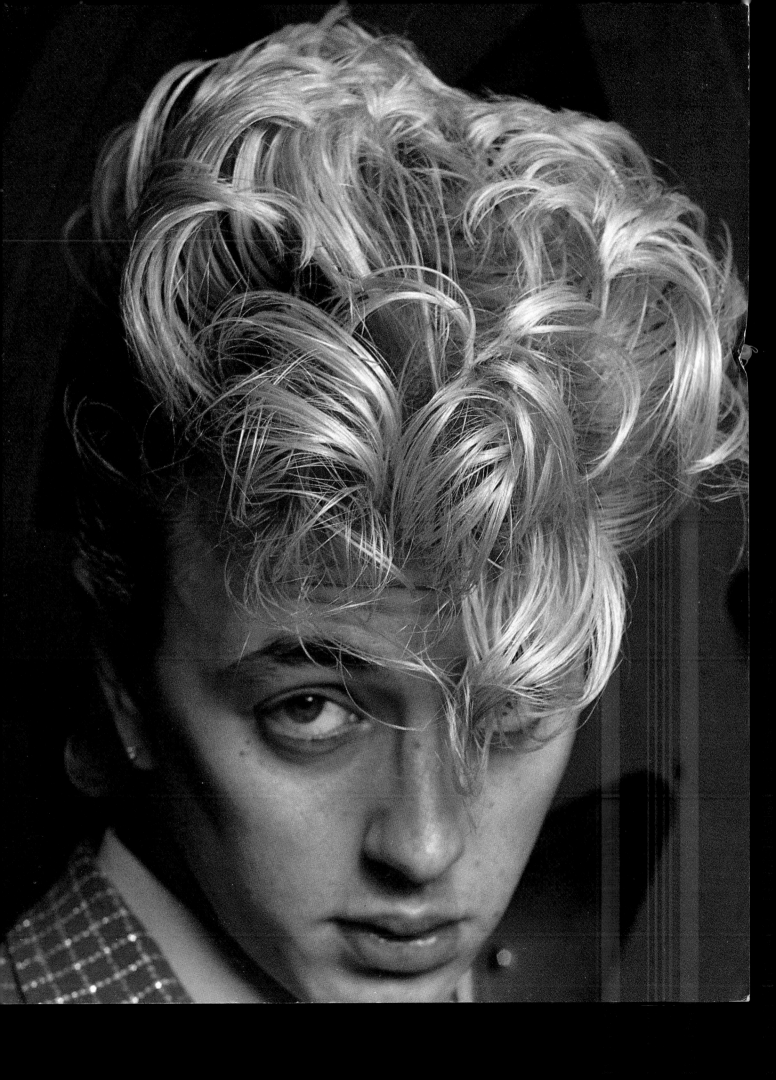

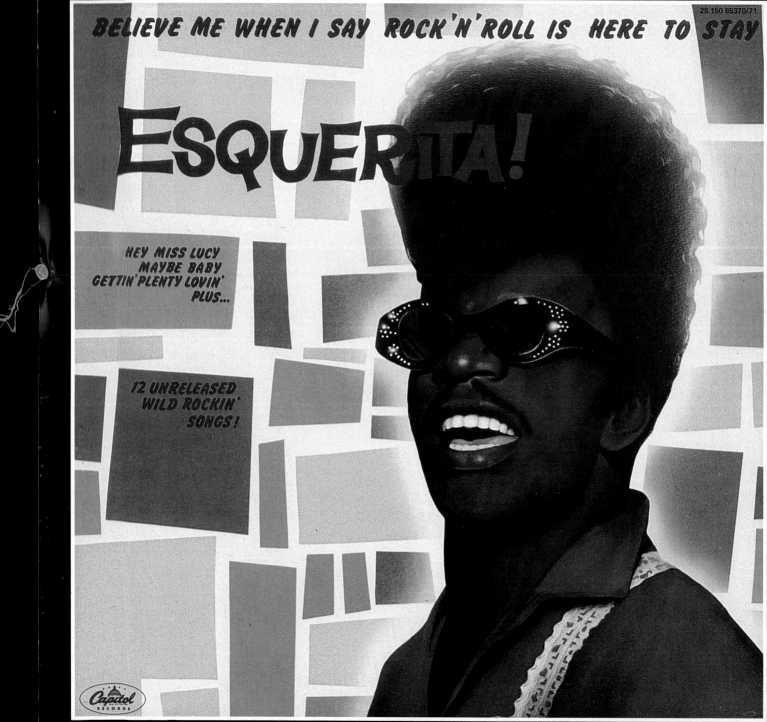

The ridiculously named Esquerita was Capitol Records' answer to Little Richard. After the success of 'the bronzed Liberace' in the late fifties, they signed Esquerita, rushing out a succession of records, most of which were bizarre, crude parodies of Richard's songs, such as 'Juicy Miss Lucy', 'Batty Over Hattie', 'Good Golly, Annie May'. Not surprisingly, Capitol were unsuccessful in their attempt at imitating one of the most exciting figures in rock 'n' roll. In only one respect did Esquerita outdo Richard: in the 'do' department. He possessed a gargantuan conk, a mile-high mass of blow-dried curls which someone once likened to the front of a '59 Continental. Born a Caucasian thirty years later, Esquerita might have been invited to swell the ranks of Sigue Sigue Sputnik. Undoubtedly he would have accepted.

esquerita!

A natural Malcolm X after he gave up the conk.

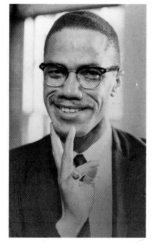

ike turner

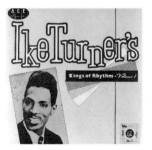

Like many black performers, Ike Turner had worn a conk or 'do' for most of his professional life. But, like Elvis Presley, he couldn't ignore The Beatles, and during the sixties turned his conk into a processed version of the mop top.

One of the most extravagant figures in rock and roll history, Little Richard (Richard Penniman) created some of the most energetic records of the fifties: wicked, pumping, orgiastic exorcisms like 'Tutti Frutti', 'Long Tall Sally' and 'Good Golly Miss Molly'. In 1959 he gave up the high life for an even higher one when he discovered religion, with which he has flirted ever since (he was once labelled as the man who put 'glossolalia in the charts'). There was almost as much of Little Richard above his neck as there was below it, and his seminal conk became his trademark, a big black penis pointing up to God.

little richard

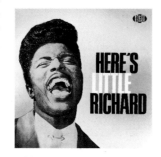

the conk

While the styles of Tony Curtis and Elvis became common currency, revamped and revived, among white youth cults, the blacks of the fifties were also making their contribution to haircut history. The story starts some decades back. The conk was born in the twenties, when American blacks first started straightening their hair to resemble Caucasian hair. Throughout the Jazz Age the desired effect was the patent leather look popularized by Cab Calloway, though during the fifties, in the wake of the massive upsurge of white r&b, black rock 'n' roll stars started wearing their conks high, in a tall 'do' – described by Penny Stallings as 'pompadours with marcelled sides and a towering cascade of waves and curls' (*Rock 'n' Roll Confidential*, 1984).

To acquire a conk took hours of painstaking straightening, using hot irons and a coagulated gunk, a 'relaxing solution'. The wet, lank hair was then combed and greased into the conk. Though it could withstand the wildest Lindy-hopping, humid weather played havoc with the conk's construction, turning the hair back to its curly state. For this reason 'do-rags' came into being, turban-like stockings which held the conks in place. These 'do-rags' have passed into legend: during the mid-eighties several gangs of Bronx b-boys developed a penchant for them (for stylistic reasons only); former hairdresser and funkadelic godfather George Clinton even immortalized the offending article in a song, 'Do The Do'.

'Malcolm X rarely exchanged any words with those Negro men with shiny, "processed" hair without giving them a nudge. Very genially: "Ahhhh, brother, the white devil has taught you to hate yourself so much that you put hot lye in your hair to make it look more like his hair." ' (Foreword to *The Autobiography of Malcolm X* by Alex Haley, 1964)

In his autobiography Malcolm X tells how he was given his first conk in Boston in 1940, shortly after buying his first zoot suit (on credit), discovering cigarettes, liquor and reefers, and learning to Lindy-hop. To avoid paying a barber the three or four dollar charge, he and a friend decided to do it themselves, first mixing up the congolene and then conking and greasing Malcolm's hair. It was a laborious process, involving a can of Red Devil lye, two eggs, two medium-sized white potatoes, a jar of Vaseline, a large bar of soap, a large-toothed comb and a fine-toothed comb, a rubber hose, a rubber apron and a pair of gloves. After painful and complicated application of the mixture, after the ironing, the drying and the combing, Malcolm X was left with his very first conk. 'My first view in the mirror blotted out the hurting. I'd seen some pretty conks, but when it's the first time, on your own head, the transformation, after a lifetime of kinks, is staggering . . . on top of my head was this thick, smooth sheen of shining red hair (X's natural colour) – real hair – straight as any white man's.'

After his conversion to the Muslim religion, Malcolm X focused attention on the way the American black man presents himself to the outside world, frowning particularly on conking, and punishing himself for his misguided, hedonistic past. He continues: 'How ridiculous I was! . . . this was my first really big step toward self-degradation when I endured all of that pain, literally burning my flesh with lye, in order to cook my natural hair until it was limp, to have it look like a white man's hair. I had joined that multitude of Negro men and women in America who are brainwashed into believing that the black people are "inferior" – and white people "superior" – that they will even violate their God-created bodies to try to look "pretty" by white standards.'

He cut off his red conk, and opted for a short close crop. During the late sixties and early seventies, when cultural insurrection played hostage to the Afro, the conk was outlawed by most blacks; it is still worn by some ageing rock 'n' rollers, though processed hair has taken many new directions in the eighties.

growing out, growing up

The late fifties saw youth culture polarise. The young teen rebels went back to highschool as doo-wop and saccharin pop stars dominated the airwaves. Elvis had joined the army, and rock'n'roll was effectively dead. Meanwhile, on the other side of town, the hipsters were stirring: art-school, ersatz existentialism and hard be-bop were the touchstones here, helping create a new breed of beatnik (*opposite*). In 1958 it was cool to be cool *and* hip to be square. A period of transition in many ways, the sixties were already here.

beatniks

If the Teds were quintessentially working class, then the beatniks, who emerged in Britain during the mid fifties, were firmly entrenched in the middle class. And whereas the Teds had been a phenomenon of group identity, rebelling against class and the *system*, a cult centred around girls, clothes, dancing and the occasional bout of violence, the beatniks were rebelling against the establishment and their *parents*.

Beatniks created the first real generation gap, questioning not only their own upbringing but also authority – government, the arms race and all bastions of middle-class affluence. Similarly, the American beat generation produced a culture of dropping out, with familiar touchstones: Ginsberg, Kerouac, Corso, Burroughs, Ferlinghetti, polo-necks, hard bop poetry, Coltrane, reefers, Juliette Greco, abstract painting, Monk, Parker, existentialism. The beat generation were basically art delinquents and the way they flouted convention was through personal and individual expression. Unlike most other expressions of youth, the boys and girls who followed the beats, the beatniks, believed the pen to be mightier than the sword. The beatniks were basically the precursors of the hippie.

Writing of this essentially middle-class tribe, Lee Gibb remarked in *The Higher Jones* (1961), 'They have replaced the American haircut by the French haircut. They have replaced high heels by low heels, low heels by no heels, and no heels by bare feet.'

Beatniks not only wanted to assume the ethnicity of black culture (white negroes), but they also wanted to expand their minds. And they managed to grow their hair whilst achieving both. As they distanced themselves from society, so a uniform of sorts began to emerge, one which wasn't meant to impress or annoy their peer groups, but to set themselves apart from society, a style which was a combination of, to quote Peter Everett, 'the French bohemian, English intellectual and US hobo.'

The Beatniks were the original back-packers, complete with straggling hair and sandals.

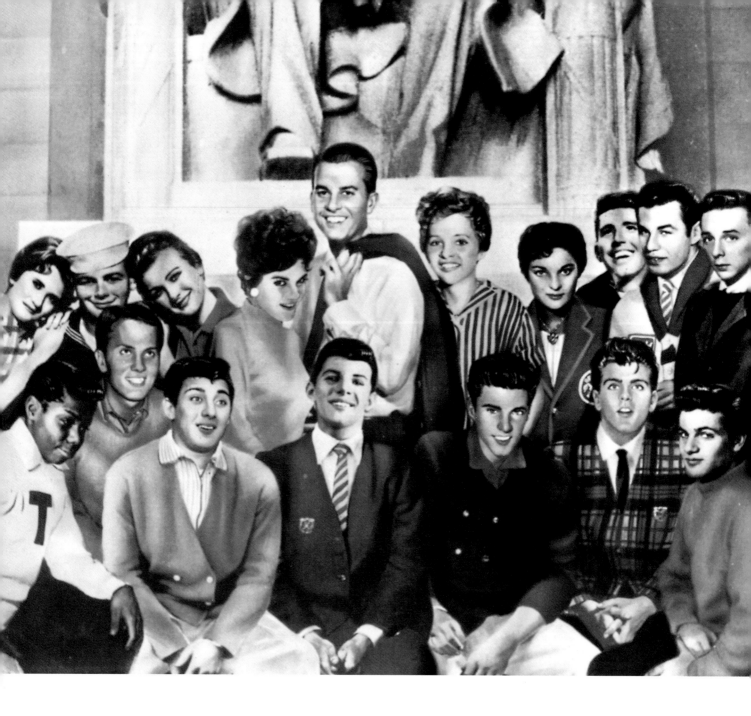

highschool

Guy Peelhaert's illustration from his book *Rock Dreams* (1973), written in conjunction with Nik Cohn, epitomizes the homogenization of the rock'n'roll myth. 'High school wasn't a musical form. It was an attitude and that attitude read: "We go to highschool. We date and go to parties and yes, we sometimes neck but no, we never pet. We also think coke and hamburgers are really neat. We wear sneakers, short skirts, highschool sweaters etc." ' The hair here is worn as inoffensively as possible, in true teen dream style. Highschool was, according to Cohn, 'an exact reflection of what white American middle-class teenagers really liked and dreamed of. Probably it was the most POP pop ever.' In their own way, the Beach Boys and the beach party films starring Frankie Avalon and Annette Funicello helped spread this cleansed interpretation of young America. Avalon and Funicello starred in seven beach movies, starting with the sanitized *Beach Party* (1960) and moving on to *Beach Blanket Bingo* and *How To Stuff A Wild Bikini*, titles which belied the movies' tame story lines.

ponytail

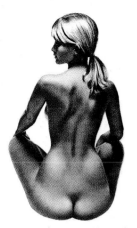

In America by the end of the forties, young girls were beginning to wear their hair in ponytails, the hair being pulled to the back of the head, tied, and then allowed to fall between the shoulders. Originally popular with country & western singers, the ponytail soon caught on with the rest of America and then the world at large. It was picked up by Teddy girls in Britain, along with baggy flared skirts, long umbrellas, alternating with the Kim Novak style of tight calf-length skirts and French plaits. It was additionally popularized by Brigitte Bardot, while a female vocal group calling themselves the Poni-tails had two Top 30 hits in 1958, *Born Too Late* and *Early To Bed*, and the following year even Picasso featured it in one of his paintings. The ponytail was identical to the hairstyle worn by the Belgic chiefs in 50 BC.

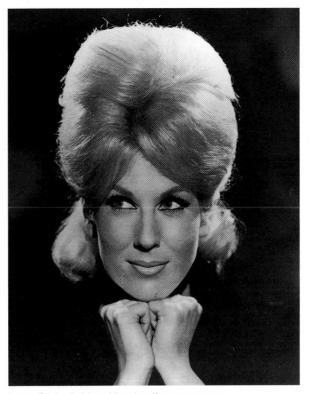

Dusty Springfield and her bouffant supreme.

bouffant

Bouffants began appearing in America during 1955, and the following year *Life* magazine reported the phenomenon: 'More exaggerated than anything seen since women hid rats in their hair at the turn of the century, this new style is a completely smooth hairdo evolved by cross-breeding last year's page-boy hair style with this spring's outsize hat. The bouffant look is basically a thick page-boy hairdo, eight to ten inches long, which has been puffed out at the sides and lacquered in place. The new hair style rules out any possibility of hats; but wearers can decorate their widespread tresses with giant bows, jewels or feathers.'

Popular with their mothers and elder sisters, in the early sixties bouffants were appropriated by the American teenager. Young girls took the style to ridiculous extremes, turning their hair into great mushroom or toadstool shapes, bubbles, even peanuts.

The shapes were similar to the grandiose designs popular with the French aristocracy in the eighteenth century and the girls of the mid twentieth century experienced the same hygiene problems. It was not unknown for high school girls to go for weeks without combing or washing their teased bouffants. In 1962 in Canton, Ohio, one young girl who hadn't attended to her great candyfloss bob for several weeks, was alarmed when her classmates noticed blood dribbling down her neck. After a thorough search by the school doctor, a nest of cockroaches was found, happy in the warm confines of the mammoth bouffant.

At a time when America was embroiled in the space race, bouffants presented a light-hearted alternative to the hordes of B-movie extra-terrestrials swarming the drive-ins with their laser guns and ill-fitting silver jumpsuits. Here were aliens right here on earth.

straight hair

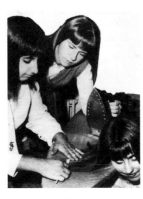

As a reaction against the backcombing of the late fifties, in the mid sixties straight hair became *de rigueur* for any young American girl. This was fine if you happened to have straight hair, but if your hair was naturally curly radical measures were called for. In the two years between 1965 and 1967 girls used dress irons to flatten their hair, usually pressing it between two brown paper bags. This often resulted in the hair having to be cut due to scorch marks.

beehive/re-hive

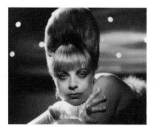

The beehive is probably the tallest haircut ever to become a cult, catching on in 1958–59, when women's hair in the United States seemed to go crazy. A beehive involved frantic backcombing, often a plastic or wire frame to provide a structure, patience, and an inordinate amount of lacquer (hairspray made technological leaps and bounds in the fifties). From 1959 until 1963 many American girls became hairhoppers, continually altering their massive beehives, strolling around like Empire State humans . . . with hair seemingly as high as a house.

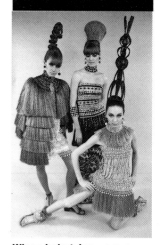

Wiggy hairstyles were a vital ingredient of Yves Saint-Laurent's collection for autumn '67.

We had a mod revival, a ska revival, a pop revival, a revival revival. The sixties didn't always look so great the second time around, but the B-52s made up for any lack of genuine caprice.

the b-52s

The B-52s took their name from sixties slang for the beehive sported by the band's girl members (Cindy Wilson and Kate Pierson), so-called because of its original resemblance to the vast B-52 bomber. Their kitsch blend of post-punk dynamics and sixties memorabilia was first heard on the 'Rock Lobster' single, released in 1978, and all their songs had titles as silly as the girls' hair: 'Quiche Lorraine', '53 Miles West of Venus', 'There's a Moon In The Sky (Called The Moon)', 'Wig'. The B-52s and their hairstyles were symptomatic of the seventies' re-use and re-appraisal of sixties pop and its associated styles. Suddenly Batman, Top Cat, beach parties, B-movies, the checkerboard twist, paper op-art, mini-skirts, pillbox hats, pantsuits, turtle-necks and Nehru jackets, Corvette Sting Rays and Barracudas, Mary Quant, flecked mohair, the Monkees and all the other peripherals of sixties US/UK kitsch-culture were hip again.

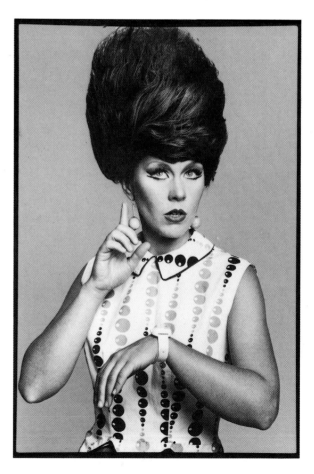

Opposite Page:
The cone was a tapering variant of the beehive.

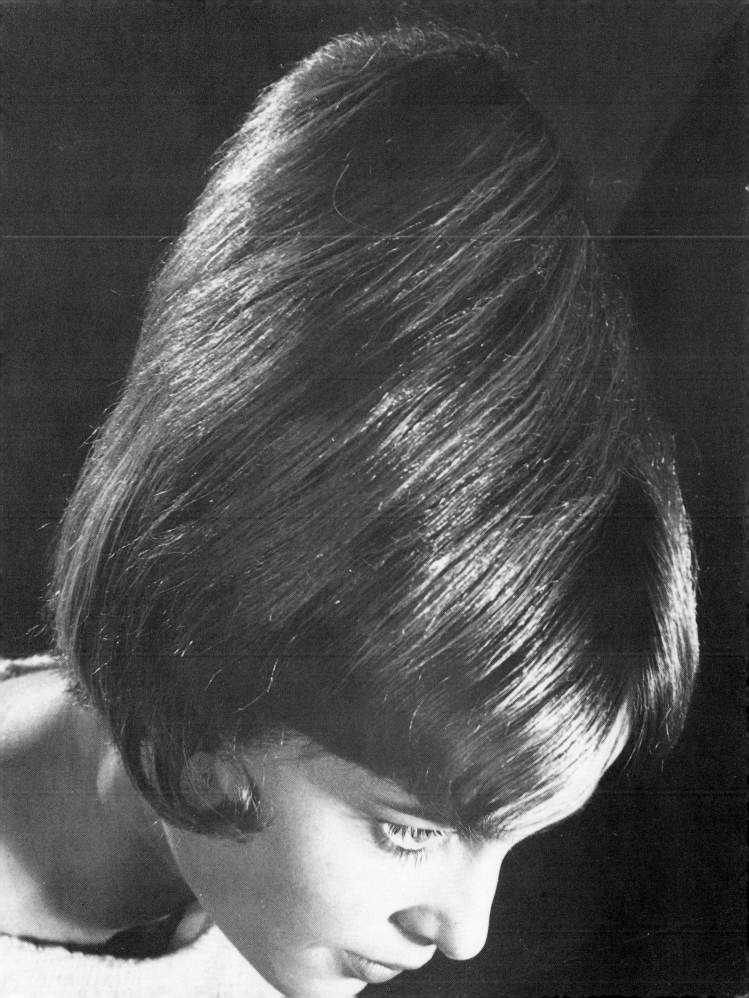

the sixties

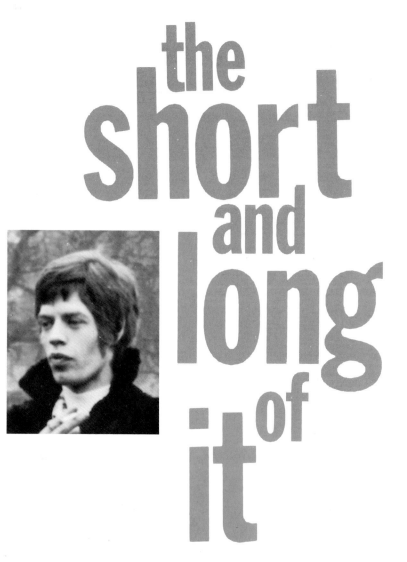

the short and long of it

In the Swinging Sixties pop culture went global. Fashion went overboard as the underground went overground, taking its emblematic hairstyles with it. This was the time of Mod, the Supremes, the Beatles, the Rolling Stones and Regency – all signposts to better times ahead. The decade was perhaps best personified by Twiggy (*opposite*), who, with her fresh features, shorn hair and happy-go-lucky temperament, became a symbol of rebellion, ambition and independence.

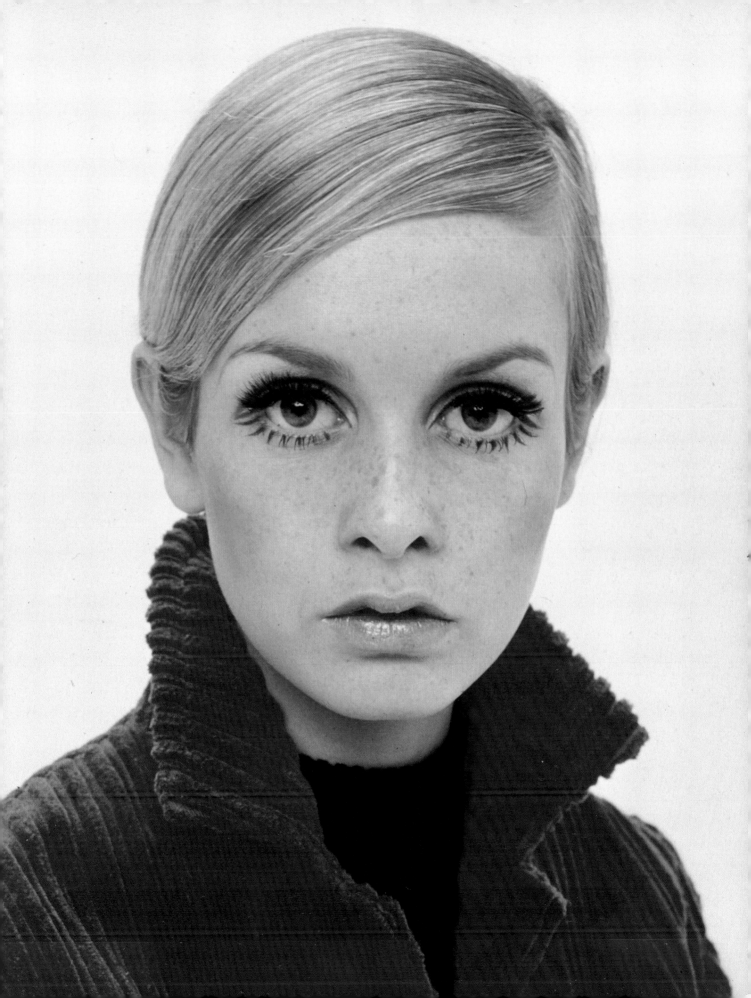

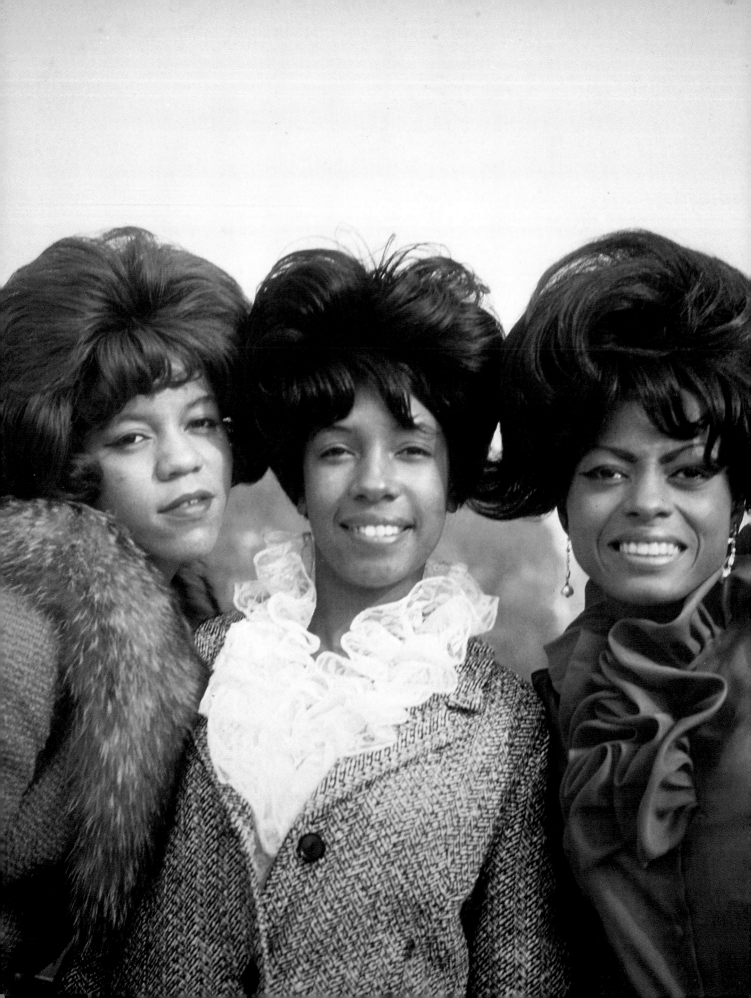

supreme time

Not only were the Supremes the first real Queens of American pop, they were also some of the first BLAPS (Black American Princesses). Whereas a lot of pop stars in the early sixties back combed their hair, teasing it into the required shape, the Supremes took the easy way out – they wore wigs. It was towards the end of 1964 – the year in which the Supremes had their first real smash hit, *Where Did Our Love Go* – that Florence Ballard, Mary Wilson and Diana Ross began accumulating wigs. After their first appearance on The Ed Sullivan Show their career took off, and finding themselves with a full calendar for the next twelve months, the girls stocked up on wigs of all shapes and sizes. 'It was easier to change wigs than to change hairstyles,' says Mary Wilson in her autobiography *Dreamgirl*. 'We each had dozens of them, all expensive, handmade human-hair pieces in a variety of styles ranging from mod-ish Vidal Sassoon cuts to high, elaborate flips. In fact, the bulk of our luggage was made up of huge wig boxes.' During this period Motown's most popular female singing group also wore padded bras, false eyelashes, hip pads, false nails and padded bottoms.

In 1964, courtesy of the Supremes, wigs suddenly became fashionable again.

twiggy

The Neasden Bambi

Many people cite the sixties as the time when 'Swinging London' fostered the notion of the classless society, or at least those people who spent their lives in society columns cite it as such. The media went pop, and London appeared to be awash with photographers, hairdressers, models, actors, singers and journalists, brightly dressed, aspirational creatures who seemed to spend all their time at photo sessions. In reality, the classless, aspirational society remained essentially a media invention.

One of the few who really did make it was Twiggy. Wearing her Mary Quant ensembles, with her tom-boy locks and big, Bambi eyes, Twiggy somehow came to represent certain aspects of the sixties: youth, ambition, self-image. The decade's youthful energy was personified in her; born Leslie Hornby in London in 1949, christened Twiggy seventeen years later when she became 'The Face Of 1966'.

With the help of her boyfriend, entrepreneur Justin de Villeneuve, Twiggy first tried to make her name as a model. She had been unsuccessful until, in 1966, she signed a contract with British fashion magazine *Woman's Mirror*. She was sent to Leonard in Mayfair's Upper Grosvenor Street to have her hair cut; but what began as a straightforward make-over turned into a haircut of epic significance.

It took over eight hours to get it right. He cut it, tinted it, cut it again, then did the highlights. 'They kept drying it,' Twiggy said, 'to see if it fell right. Those short haircuts have to be absolutely precise. The back was just an inch long, with a little tail, and the front very smooth. I thought it was marvellous.' So did everyone else. Photographer Barry Lategan did a session with her, a print from which Leonard put in his salon window, where it was spotted by the *Daily Express* fashion editor Dierdre McSharry.

That paper subsequently called Twiggy 'The Face Of 1966', and her own era was well and truly born. The close-cropped light brown hair became synonymous with the whole sixties look (the Quant miniskirts, Op Art boots, etc), a haircut *Newsweek* called 'the year's most radiant and evocative new image'.

the mop top

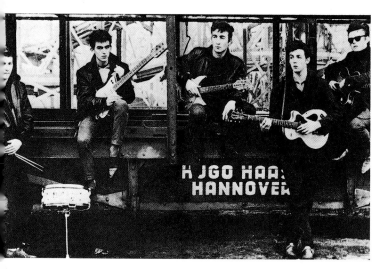

The Beatle cut didn't involve greasing or pomade, and ushered in a new period of completely dry hairdressing. At the tail-end of the fifties the Beatles had worn grease emphatically; in fact in 1959 they looked like any other undernourished, floundering rock 'n' roll group – five skinny boys with pallid complexions clad in leather jackets and unwashed quiffs.

In these fledgling years they were just another bunch of loud-mouthed hopefuls, until they met Brian Epstein. Later, it would be Epstein's job to turn them into palatable pop fodder, which he successfully did, with hip collarless jackets, Chelsea boots and cheesey grins. By then, the Beatles had already acquired their first major gimmick, the haircut which would become their trademark, courtesy of a young German girl called Astrid Kirchherr, a model, photographer, and sometime hairdresser.

The Beatles in Hamburg, Germany, before the haircut which would help change their lives. Pete Best, George Harrison, John Lennon, Paul McCartney and Stuart Sutcliffe.

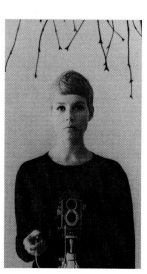

Astrid Kirchherr – the girl who shaped the sixties.

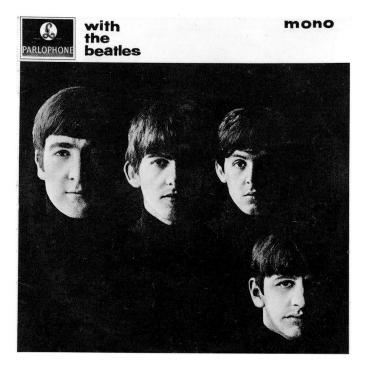

with the beatles mono
PARLOPHONE

With The Beatles **LP sleeve from 1963, one of the most famous mop-top icons, the harsh black and white photography emphasizing their sinking fringes.**

the beatle wig

The Beatle wig, once enormously popular, and still sought after as a piece of kitsch pop memorabilia. In America in 1964 Beatle wigs were manufactured in their thousands, and strangely, considering their popularity and the longevity of the Beatles as a marketable product, the wigs are now extremely scarce. To the uninitiated the wigs still look like miniature black nylon hearthrugs.

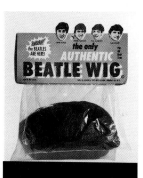

those beatle bangs

Stuart Sutcliffe, the phenomenally good-looking fifth Beatle who later died of a brain tumour, was pursued by the German beauty while the band were living and performing in Hamburg during 1960, eventually becoming her boyfriend. She was instrumental in the transformation of the group from shabby nobodies to stylish contenders. She introduced them to leather trousers, and, via Sutcliffe, the infamous mop top.

One day in Hamburg she combed Sutcliffe's greased 'cockade' forward, and cut it into a French style – a variation of the French Caesar cut, a modified fifteenth-century style with long bangs completely covering the forehead. Sutcliffe was the butt of many jokes from the other Beatles when he turned up to play at the Kaiserkeller Club that night, his hair combed straight forward, not a hint of grease in sight. Later he swept it back into a typical Elvis style before going on stage, but twenty-four hours later he turned up with his Beatle fringe, and from then on kept it.

George Harrison soon started wearing his hair this way too, though it took another five months before John and Paul followed suit. Pete Best never adopted the look, and this is often given as the reason why he was asked to leave the group! Enormously popular, enormously influential, the Beatle cut was copied the world over. It was also the first mass market appearance of 'long hair'; it hadn't really been acceptable for men to wear their hair over their ears since the First World War.

The mop top caused considerable controversy, with many church organizations seeing it as a catalyst for world disorder. President Lyndon Johnson even made a point of asking the boys to go get themselves a trim. They caused a furore, though the lovable Mop Tops' orthodox and almost boy-next-door demeanour made it hard for them to be outcast. By the mid sixties the Beatles had become part of the very fabric of British and global life. Even Elvis Presley, try as he might, couldn't ignore the Beatles, making a concession to Beatlemania (albeit somewhat after the event) when he exchanged his bible-black wedge for Beatle bangs in a 1969 movie called *Change of Habit*, the last of his thirty-one excursions into film.

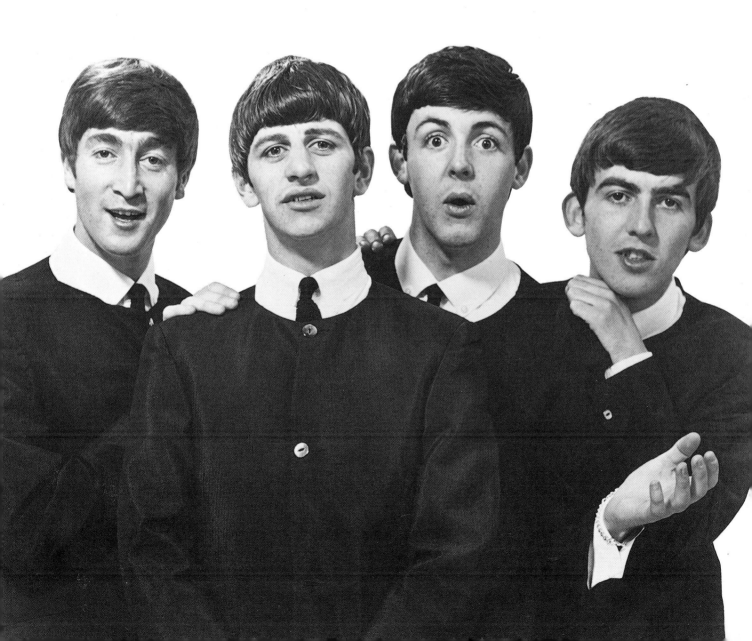

mods

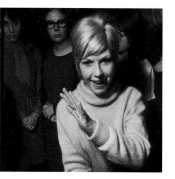

Homely girl: suburban mod extraordinaire.

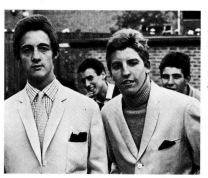

A gathering of typical mods, en route for either the Scene, the Flamingo, the Mecca, the Marquee, the Palais or the Locarno: goin' to a go-go.

the italian job and the french connection

The original modernists (named after their favourite music, modern jazz) emerged at the very beginning of the sixties; many of them came from middle-class Jewish families in north London. They were obsessed by clothes and looking sharp; a welcome relief after the gauche activities of the Teds, the modernist way of life was soon adopted by working class youth in general, and Britain had a major sub-culture on its hands.

Mods were infatuated with clothes and paid an obsessive attention to detail, loving the clean lines of well cut trousers or shirts. Smug in the knowledge that they owned the right jacket with the right side vents, mods were the first teenage dandies, and their continental attire (borrowed from the Italians and the French) was the complete opposite of all that lumbering crape and drape of the fifties. This was very much a male tribe, and girls were placed fifth in the mod priority list, below clothes, hair, drugs and transport. Mods were completely narcissistic: 'Gradually the new attitude caught on, the notion of dressing out of self-love rather than rebellion and, by 1962, there were enough converts to make a sect, which was called mod.' (Nik Cohn).

Living life to the full, mods took fast drugs, spent their spare afternoons shopping, their evenings posing and their nights dancing. A mod had a bigger wardrobe than the rest of his family put together, and often changed clothes three or four times a day. He liked black music, Italian scooters and French haircuts.

In *Mods!* (1979), the definitive work on the subject, Richard Barnes writes: 'Italian haircuts had come in about 1960. Not all barbers could do an Italian haircut, as most of them still simply cut men's hair rather than styling it, but for about 6/– (as opposed to the normal 2/6d) you could get the "Perry Como" cut. The style had a different ,"dry" look because kids had no oil or grease on it and in those days it wasn't easy to get out of the barbers without him rubbing some sort of oil into your hair.'

Then came the shorter French college boy cut, the two inch crew-cut, the French crew and the French crop – a college cut with a higher parting.

The seminal mod haircut, however, was the back-combed look, with a short half-parting high on the head, with the rest gaining height at the back. Richard Barnes again: 'Special "bobble combs" for backcombing became standard equipment and guys started lacquering hair to keep it in position. Hair could be raised two or three inches with practice, effort and a backcomb. Rod Stewart had the most far-out backcombed hair I ever saw. His hair was longer than most mods, and it rose up from just in front of his crown to it seemed about six inches in height.' Mod girls' hair changed from bouffants to very straight hair . . . the two styles were either parted in the centre, chin length, or with a heavy deep fringe. One of the most famous mod girl styles was the Cleopatra look worn by television pop presenter Cathy McGowan. (Such was the importance of the mod locks that seminal mod clone band The Who were originally going to be called The Hair.) Mods were inclined to frequent nightclubs and dancehalls six nights a week. The other night was reserved for the ritual washing of the hair.

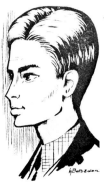

October 25, 1963, HAIRDRESSERS' JOURNAL — MAGAZINE SECTION 25

How to Cut the New French Line

THIS is a classic interpretation of the new Club line for men, launched by the French men's hairdressing *Syndicat*. It is quiet and sober in its design but smart and groomed enough for any age group.

The hair is a little longer than in most recent men's lines. It is not so much thinned by the razor as carefully refined.

Fig. 1. After having put in the parting (1) make a division through the hair just above the temple (A).

By making a second division a little lower (B), one can shield the " shoulder " meshes which correspond to the area of the greatest volume in the finished style.

The base of the sides is thinned vertically according to the shape of the head.

Fig. 2. The back and nape hair is reduced with the razor, the scissors being used to control only the extreme points.

All the overlapping meshes on the top of the head must be gone over again very lightly with the razor to obtain a good blending of the points, while retaining fullness just below the parting.

Fig. 3. In dressing out, secure volume at the sides by taking a small round styling brush and, having determined the thickness of the mesh (1) place the brush at the root (2). Lift the hair with a turning movement while directing the hot air jet from the dryer on to top of the head (3).

Fig. 4. To obtain a natural volume at the level of the parting, force the roots a little with the comb *against* the natural direction of the hair growth.

Except for smoothing the hair, take care not to flatten the volume which has been achieved.

by

Fernand Gautier

Member of the Syndicat de la Haute Coiffure Masculine and of the Comite Artistique ile la Coiffure Francaise

COVERING MESH

THINNING

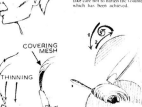

Right: **Mod remake/remodel: mod approximates photographed in 1986 for an exhibition on teenage consumerism at The Boilerhouse gallery in London.**

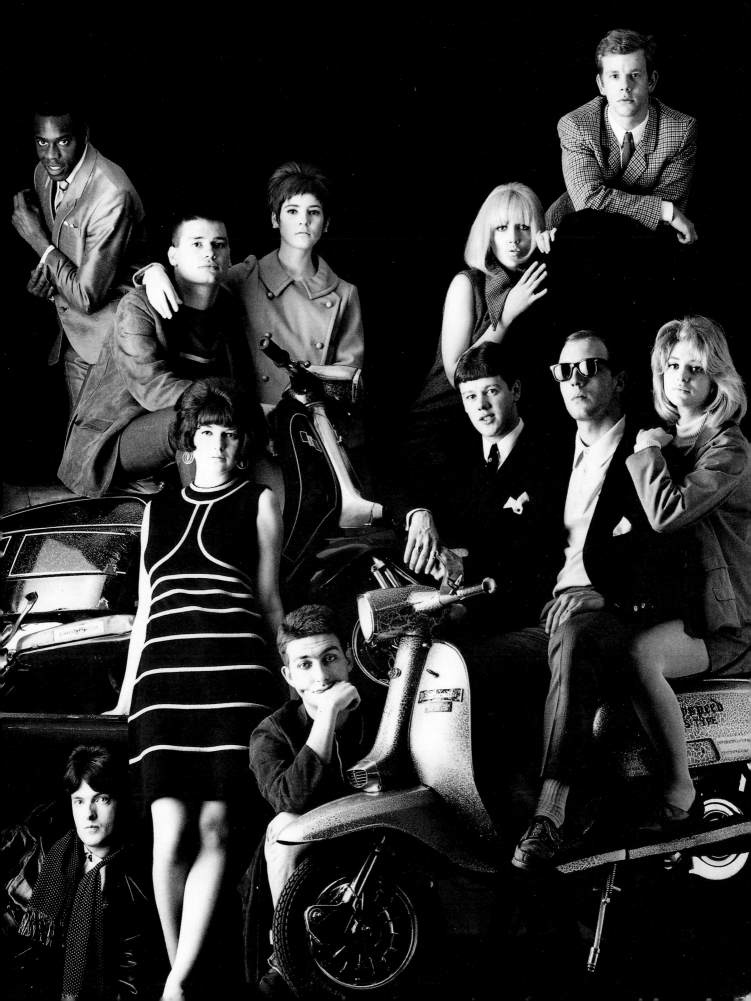

back to the stone age

Subversion! Whereas the Beatles were thought of as lovable mop tops, the Rolling Stones were regarded with the utmost suspicion. Their records were louder, their dress more extreme, their hair longer, their language ugly. They also seemed completely uninterested in the entertainment business, because to Brian Jones, Mick Jagger, Keith Richards, Bill Wyman and Charlie Watts business meant gutbucket r&b.

To the public they seemed dangerous, and this was the first time since the mid fifties that pop music had taken on deviant connotations. The Stones' hair was, to quote Nik Cohn (*Awopbobaloobop Alopbamboom*, 1969), '... used as a kick in the teeth, as insult and ridicule heaped on every drabness of the system; hair as symbolic of sex, of energy; hair almost as religion. When one grew one's hair long like the Stones ... it was done as a banner, a battle-sign, and first it spread to other pop groups, the ex-art school, rhythm 'n' blues bands like the Kinks and the Pretty Things; and then to their followers; and then to the lump of modish, discontented young.'

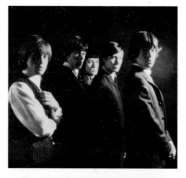

Would you let your daughter go out with a Rolling Stone? The answer was always no. Here are the Stones as they appeared on the cover of their first, eponymous British LP in 1964.

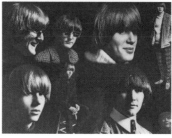

The Byrds, exploiters of folk-rock, with the look of 1966. *Turn! Turn! Turn!*

regency

After mod and before psychedelia there was Regency: in 1966, after two years rampant dandyism in London, the media caught up with the sartorial extravagances of the city and christened the whole 'scene' 'Regency'. Carnaby Street soon followed suit, filling Soho with 'Buttons and Beaux', copycat dandies with more money than sense (at the time there was even a less than successful pop singer called Beau Brummell).

Midway between mod and the madness which was to follow, Regency hair was a mirror, almost, of the way people were wearing their hair on the West Coast of America: long, but not that long; untidy, but not that untidy. True to form, those very same pop stars brought back the Regency look, wholesale, oblivious to the implications.

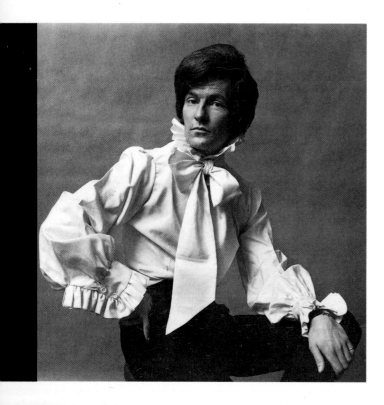

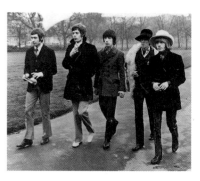

Right: Here, strolling through Hyde Park in February 1967, the Rolling Stones parade their own approximation of both Regency style, and 1966 hair. Post-yob, pre-yippie.

Left: Patrick Lichfield pictured himself as a dandy in this 1968 self-portrait.

vidal sassoon

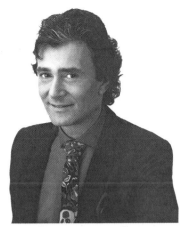

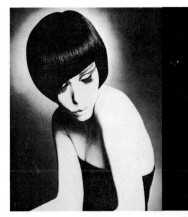

Above far right: A typical Sassoon hairstyle from 1966.
Above right: Vidal Sassoon.
Far right: The asymmetric Isadora cut by Vidal Sassoon in 1968.
Right: Sassoon's five point cut, the revolutionary geometric cut of 1964.
Below: Nancy Kwan in 1963.

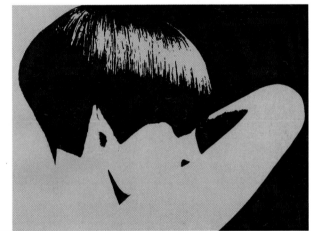

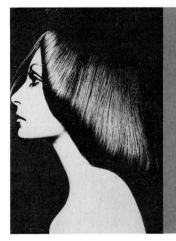

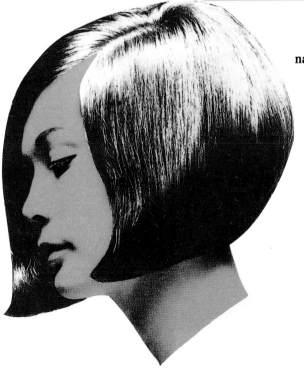

'The big name in hairdressing this week is Vidal Sassoon. It is a name that might become bigger in the years to come.' (*Hairdressers' Journal*, 3 July 1958)

Borrowing the style of twenties film actress Louise Brooks, London hairdresser Vidal Sassoon revolutionized womens' hairdressing in 1963 by re-inventing the bob. Before the bob, hair had been worn UP, either in bouffants or beehives, but the loose flat hair of the Sassoon look signalled the beginning of a completely new era.

In Vidal Sassoon's own words: 'In 1963 Mary Quant came to me with a problem... "Vidal, I'm sick to death of all these chignons we've been using at the shows. I know we can't have hair hanging down over the models' shoulders, but surely there is some other way to keep it away from the clothes?" "Sure," I said, "you could cut the whole damn lot off!" I tried the cut out on Mary first, cutting her hair like she cut material. No fuss. No ornamentation. Just a neat swinging line.

'It caught on faster than any line I had done before or have done since. Much of the credit for encouraging the general public to accept it, however, must go to Nancy Kwan. I was asked to cut Nancy's hair for her role in *The Wild Affair*, and Terence Donovan was brought in to take that now famous picture for *Vogue*.' Throughout the sixties Sassoon would continually experiment with his bob, creating many successful mutants in the process.

towards the seventies

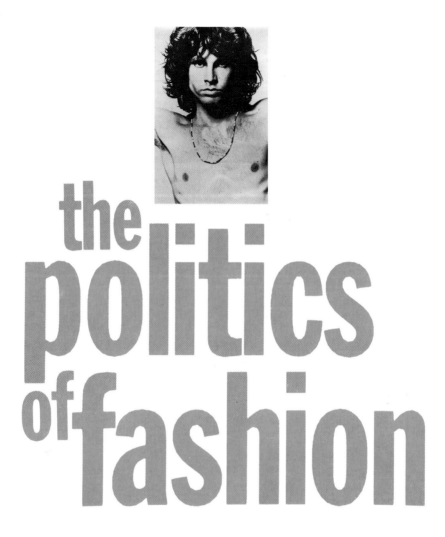

the politics of fashion

By 1967 the hippy movement was coming to a head. The world was awash with freaks, from the truly committed hedonists to the weekend hippies (with their tailor-made wigs). Here was born the alternative society, where your badge was your hair – and the longer the better. Music and fashion were entwined in a desperate scramble for meaning – which often only resulted in over-indulgence and pretentiousness. But things were changing: sexual militancy and musical expediency were just around the corner. Robert Plant (*opposite*) and Led Zeppelin would help see to that.

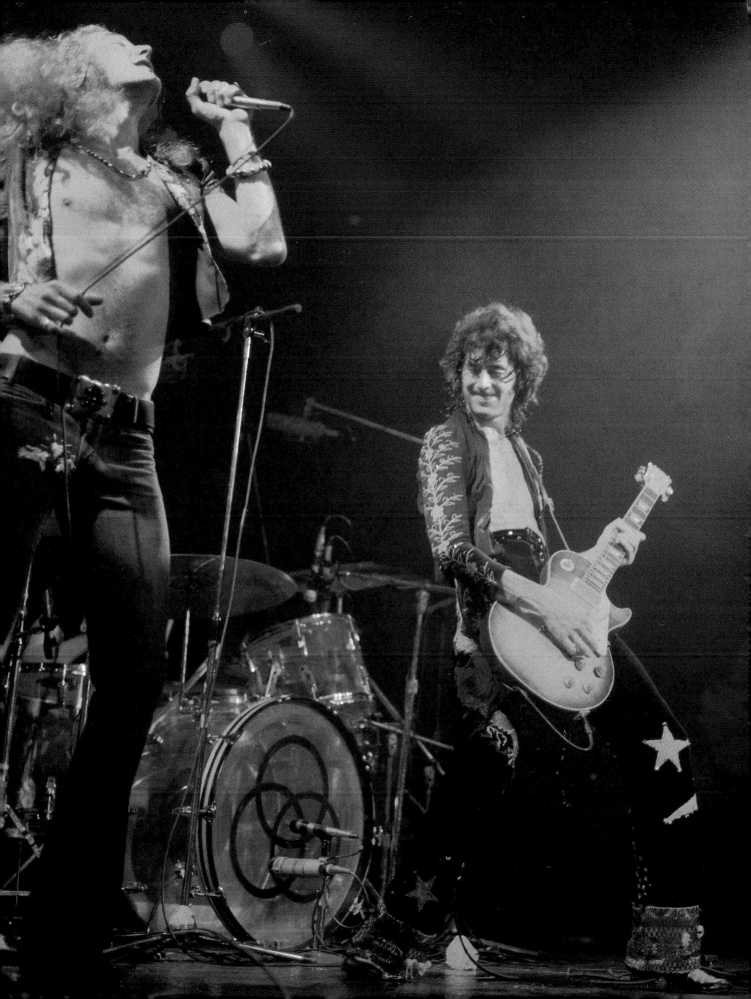

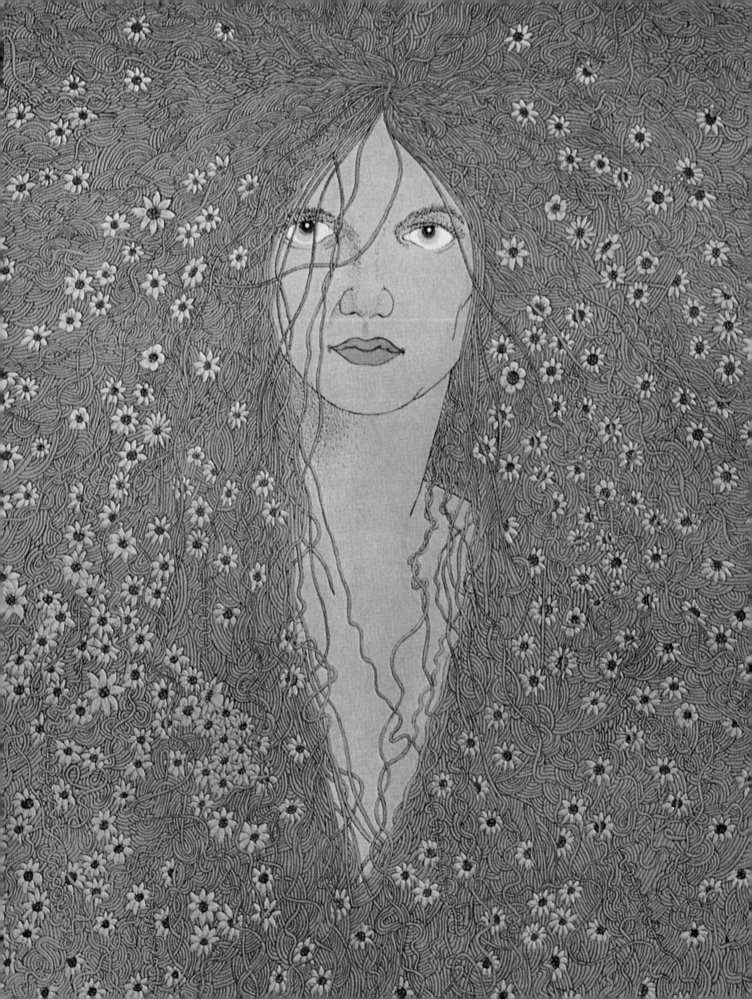

hair!

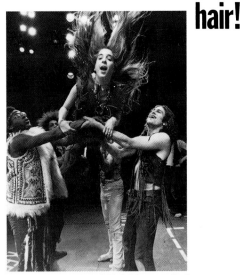

The flowing locks of *Hair!* the musical.

long hair

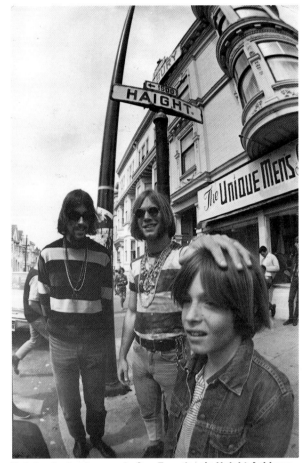

Hair beginning to grow in San Francisco's Haight-Ashbury.

Hair had been getting longer ever since the Beatles. Not only did long hair reflect a change in fashions but a change in attitudes. The love generation wanted a little more than regular pay cheques, a good car and a life in suburbia. In fact, it wanted a lot more. The unrest which had stirred the beats and their followers in the fifties was now manifesting itself all across North America, as those teenagers who had seen the light began dropping out.

revolution! evolution!

Long hair began to take on deviant status, as the connotations were not just drugs, sex and rock'n'roll, but a complete rejection of conventional social mores. It was a symbolic return to seemingly truer spiritual values, a rejection of mechanization and the rat race. Once again hair became a sign of rebellion, immediately apparent in a song like 'Almost Cut My Hair' by Crosby Stills & Nash. Society was worried: in 1968 at the Brien McMahon High School in Norwalk, Connecticut, fifty-three male students were suspended because of the length of their hair, and the town also boasted a billboard which read 'Beautify America – Get a Haircut!' Similar paranoia spread across North America, as the media got ready for a counter-cultural revolution.

Initially, San Francisco's Haight-Ashbury area became the focus for this new drug culture, a holy grail for thousands of disillusioned kids all over the States. Here, conflicting notions of the counter-culture expressed themselves – Ken Kesey's Merry Pranksters, Emmett Grogan's notorious Diggers and many others toyed with cornership utopia. For a while, from 1965 through 1966, times really did seem to be changing, and the San Franciscan longhairs created their own little bit of bohemia; but predictably, the parasites and conmen moved in, helping to create the highly spurious Summer of Love, a marketing ploy engineered to help sell bulk purchases of

flower power

Bradbury Thompson's *Flower Child* (opposite), a poster much reproduced in the late sixties, shows how the graphics of the hippy movement shared with their Art Nouveau predecessors an obsession with long hair.

but predictably, the parasites and conmen moved in, helping to create the highly spurious Summer of Love, a marketing ploy engineered to help sell bulk purchases of hippy paraphernalia, which was soon available from every market stall and trendi-deli in the area. 'Hashbury' was soon awash with LSD shamen, the psychedelic bums who led their apostles into uncharted regions of the human psyche and who, instead of altering society, in many cases succeeded only in altering their own minds.

The Summer of Love became, to paraphrase Emmett Grogan, 'one big fashion show', just a love hoax inside a giant Rick Griffin hologram. Many of these original hippies were really trying to create an alternative society, but only after convincing themselves they were from the oppressed class, which most of them certainly were not. Some, leaving their campuses or suburban dream homes flocked to Haight-Ashbury or New York's Lower East Side, proclaiming themselves to be the 'new niggers' – though for many the Summer of Love was the dawning of a new era, for others it was nothing but an 'adventure of poverty' (hippy was originally black slang for a weekend hipster). But long hair did change the way men appeared to the world. Suddenly it was okay to be weedy and thin; if you couldn't look tough, you could look weird . . . and in 1966 looking weird was better. Having hair somehow alleviated the traumas of teenage existence – it let you out.

The development of the Afro can be linked to the rise of militant black politics in the mid sixties. In the black movement there had always been a split between the integrationist civil rights movement, led by Martin Luther King, involving organizations like the NAACP and the Urban League, and the separatist wing which included Malcolm X and the Black Muslims.

Militants criticized the old civil rights leaders for their integrationist stance and style; with their suits and short hair, they were labelled 'Toms'. Hair and style came to be means of political expression, and the first real Afros began to emerge, with young blacks – at first mainly students – picking up on the political and stylistic signals.

black panther, black pride

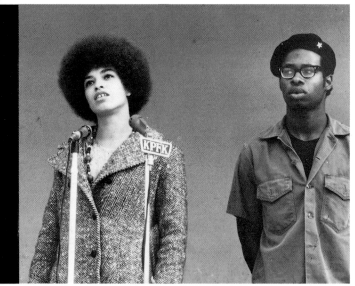

The high-rise Afro belonging to feminist and race relations campaigner Angela Davis was a symbolic constituent of her threatening aura.

In 1967 the *New York Times* carried reports on black campus revolts, noting not just the political action but also the look. They quoted a member of the Afro American Students Union at the University of California as saying: 'We decided to remember our African heroes, our American heroes and our culture. We decided to stop hating ourselves, trying to look like you, bleaching our hair, straightening our hair. In high school I used to hold my big lip in.'

Nineteen-sixty-eight was the year the Afro came to prominence in the States. Sly Stone toured America and Britain with a huge wild cut, and James Brown also changed his style from his previous elaborate conk. Records celebrating black pride made the charts; Brown's 'Say it Loud, I'm Black And I'm Proud' and Nancy Wilson's 'Black is Beautiful'.

This was also the year that the Black Panthers were at their most visible and influential. From their formation in 1966 they had understood stylistic politics and their black leather-clad urban guerrilla image was one of the most effective manifestations of black power. They advocated the Afro unequivocally, and suddenly there was an equation between how long your Afro was and how black you were. Tom Wolfe, in *Radical Chic*, says 'Christ, if those panthers don't know how to get it all together, as they say, the tight pants, the tight black turtle necks, the leather coats, cuban shades, Afros. But real Afros, not the ones that have been shaped and trimmed like a topiary hedge and sprayed until they have a sheen like acrylic wall to wall, but like funky, natural, scraggly . . . wild.'

'Can you begin to get the guts to develop criteria of beauty for black people? Your nose is boss, your lips are thick, you are black and you are beautiful. Can you begin to do it so that you are not ashamed of your hair?' (Stokely Carmichael)

Oddly, not all Panthers wore their hair in the Afro style – it was difficult for Panther leaders to grow Afros since they spent a lot of time in gaol, where their hair was cut. There was also the problem of fitting an Afro into a military-style beret.

The Afro was now the most distinctive image of black pride, part of the counter-cultural iconography of the late sixties. It was also a crucial part of the whole Pan-African Renaissance, along with clothes like dashikis, bubas, djellabas, kaftans and agbadas. Campaigns were mounted to teach African history to black students and blacks were encouraged to learn Swahili as an aid to establishing identity. The Afro, as its name suggests, was slotted into the project and provided another link with Africa. It has been said that there was an actual African precedent for the Afro in the form of the so-called 'African Bush' (a kind of short natural), but even if this was so, it was certainly no competitor to the fully fledged Afro.

The Afro invoked a kind of mythological, imaginary Africa: there was nothing particularly African or natural about the cut. It required frequent combing and, in some cases, trips to the hairdresser to get the shape right. In fact, when it reached Africa, the Afro tended to be worn by rich élites who wanted to look Western, modern, even American. Tanzania went so far as to ban the Afro, denouncing it as cultural neo-colonialism.

By 1972 the radical charge of the Afro had evaporated, and by the following year it had become slotted into a ghetto stereotype of superbad style and slangy, street-corner attitudes.

the natural

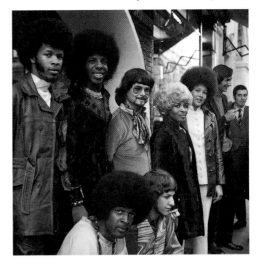

Prior to the emergence of the Afro, in the late fifties some hipsters, militants and students began wearing the natural, a wiry, short, unprocessed cut, as a reaction against conking. It caused a stir all of its own. In his book *Revolutionary Suicide*, black activist Huey Newton remembers how inspirational the style was in 1959: 'One of my friends at Oakland City College was Richard Thorne. Richard was a very tall, very black fellow who even then, prior to the "Black Cultural Revolution", wore his hair in a natural. His appearance caused awe in some people and frightened others.' Variations on the natural were sported in the same period by teenage gangs in the northern ghettoes. The most influential seems to have been the 'ranger bush' worn by the Rangers gang in Chicago. This was a thick bush of hair on top, tapered on a slant towards the back and cut close on the sides. Gang members told gullible sociologists that they developed the style because it helped to cushion the beatings they took from the cops.

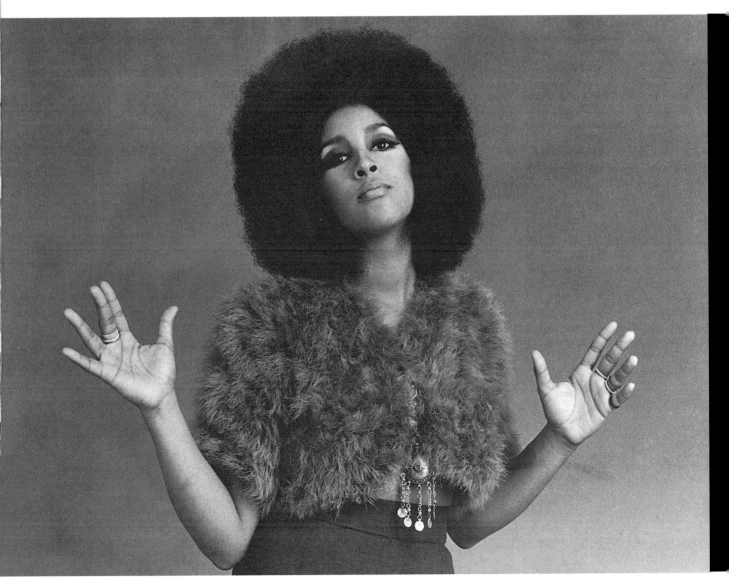

Media fascination with the Afro accelerated with the opening of the musical *Hair!* in London during September 1968 (it had opened on Broadway on 28 April), when Marsha Hunt's bouffant cut formed the basis for a poster campaign. 'I was only a member of the chorus, but I got a lot of publicity because of my hair,' she said in *Melody Maker* in May 1969.

rug alert

john stephen's wigs

In Britain, fashion designer John Stephen created a line of 'groovy' wigs. Stephen was an enormously influential figure in the London fashion world during the sixties – at one point owning nine retail outlets in Carnaby Street, London's 'peacock alley' – so his male wigs were taken quite seriously when they appeared, especially by those men who indulged in wearing Stephen's suede waistcoats, kaftan jackets, crushed velvet flared trousers and pink shirts (unheard of at the time).

In America, men of all ages welcomed wigs, as having short hair quickly became such a social stigma. There were all kinds of wigs, and a few men with long hair wore short-haired wigs to go to work in. By 1970, due to the ubiquity of wig-wearing, and a diminishing 'embarrassment factor', men were trying them on and buying them openly at beauty salons and department stores. It didn't last: attitudes towards long hair eventually changed so much that wigs became superfluous.

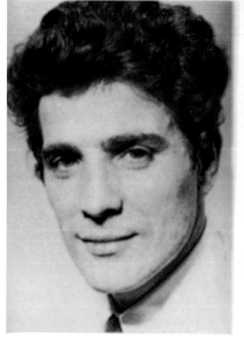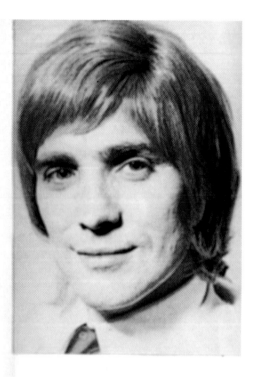
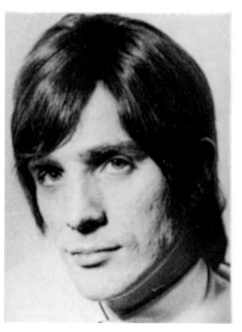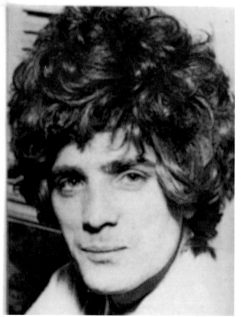

John Stephen is pictured here with his own, quite short hair (top left), and three of his wigs.

the afro wig

First introduced into the States in 1968, the Afro wig provided an opportunity for those uncertain of black revolutionary claims to evade political choice by wigging out at weekends. It was also an aid for potentially compromised black entertainers. Diana Ross appeared at the London Royal Variety Show in 1968 sporting an Afro wig, making several 'controversial' statements – quoting Martin Luther King onstage and Stokely Carmichael backstage. The wig also allowed vulnerable political institutions to make concessions without losing face. American prison authorities insisted that all black inmates should have their Afros shorn, but then let them wear wigs. In fact, the Afro wig worn by Black Panther George Jackson in San Quentin provided the guards there with the perfect reason for shooting him in 1971. They claimed he had a 9mm automatic pistol beneath it.

An Afro wig was a popular accessory during the late sixties.

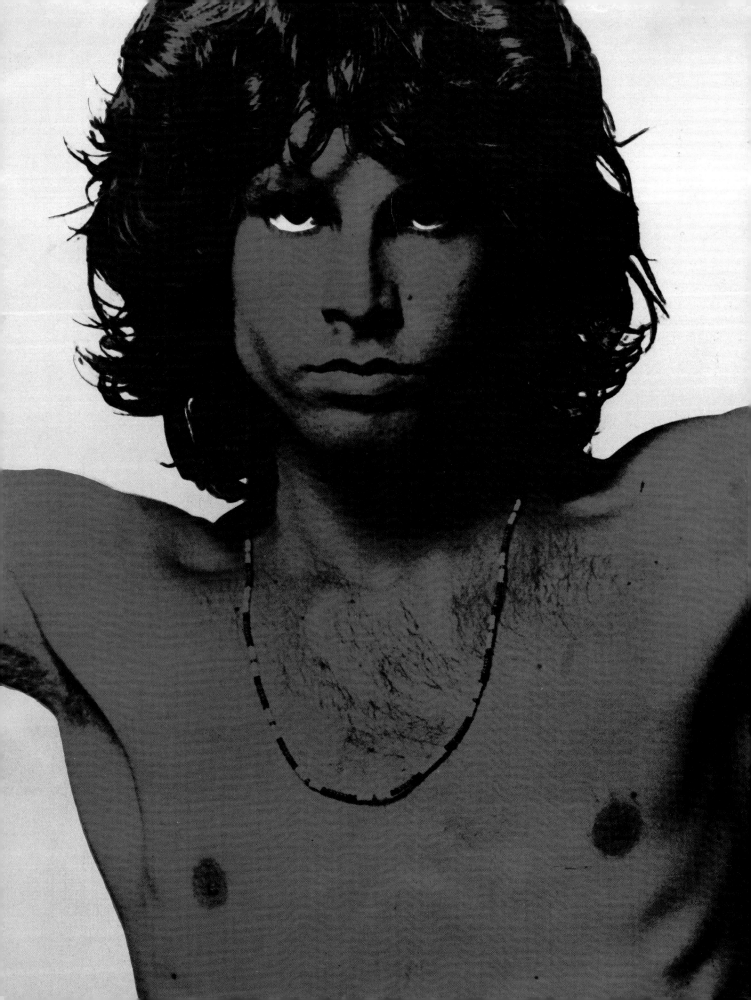

the mane chance

Towards the end of the sixties, the time of mass student insurrection and a disillusionment with hippy culture, long hair – for men at least – began to take on different connotations. No longer was it considered earthy, spiritual or sensitive. Instead, it became stroppy and macho. Not ethereal, not feminine, but virile, sweaty, male.

Characteristic of this shift was the emerging popularity of such groups as Led Zeppelin, the

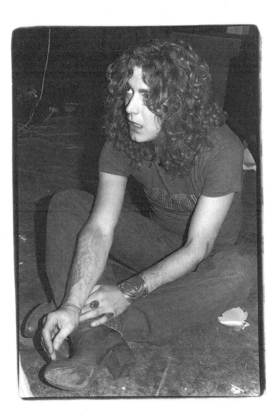

original Monsters of Rock. Zeppelin were like born-again Vikings, their rape-and-pillage musings camouflaged in mystical rhetoric. And to match their neanderthal rock they wore neo-neanderthal hair, great manes of messy machismo. Led Zeppelin were big, bad, and thoroughly business-minded; though what the establishment couldn't figure out was how these outriders of Hippy-Satan had become so darn popular and so darn rich so damn quickly!

But what they couldn't understand they learned to live with. In 1972, though longhairs still had trouble getting into Disneyland, they had gained some semblance of respect in the hotels of Los Angeles. In the foyer of the Continental Hyatt House on Sunset Boulevard a framed sign appeared depicting a typically tatty and downbeat longhair; underneath was the inscription: 'Treat this man with respect, he may have just sold a million records.'

**Led Zeppelin's
Robert Plant contemplates
his feminine machismo.**

Left: **The iconographic
photograph of the seminal
sixties 'New Man', the
Dionysiac Jim Morrison,
taken by Joel Brodsky.
Morrison's hair
represented both sexual
potency and poetic
sensitivity. Some thought of
him as Samson, and that if
his hair was cut . . .**

the seventies

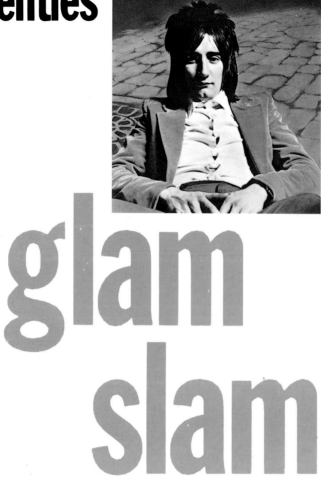

glam slam

By the time the sixties were over, virtually every length of hair had been seen, from Beatles bangs to flowing hippy locks. After such a parade, almost anything was possible: and it came in extremes, from the skinheads to the purveyors of overt male glamour. In the postcard portrait of Bryan Ferry (*opposite*) his 'elephant trunk' quiff heralded a decade of self-consciousness, a slap in the face for the idealism of the late sixties which had never taken too kindly to the narcissistic, shallow and dreadfully fickle world of fashion.

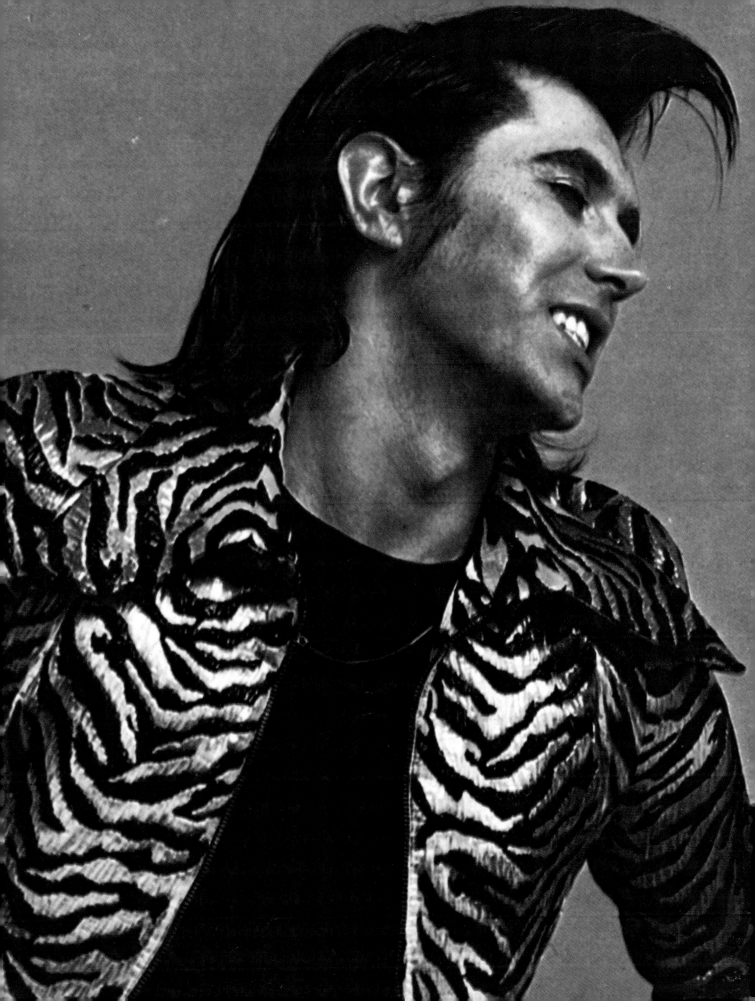

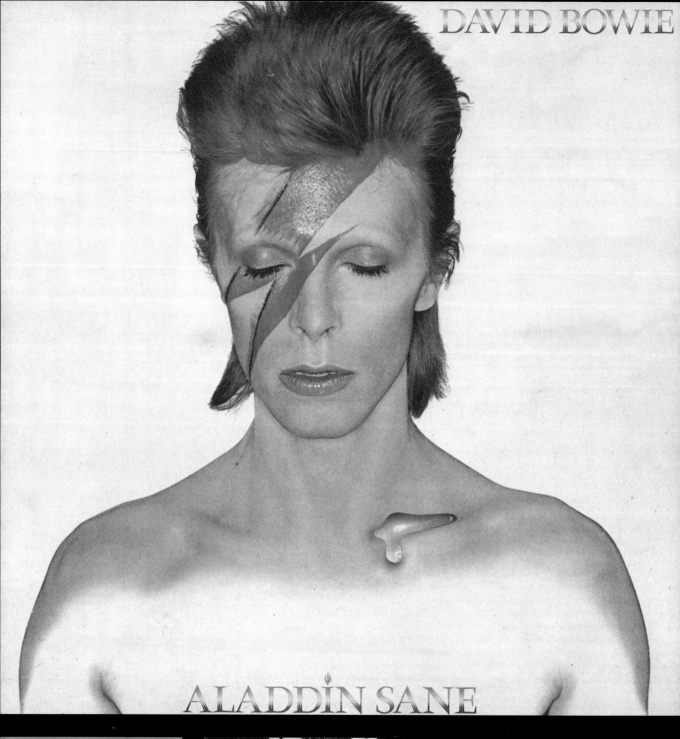

DAVID BOWIE

ALADDIN SANE

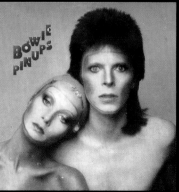

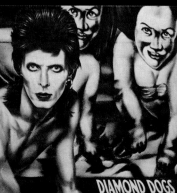

david bowie

Androgyny, self-obsession, and the return of the idol

By 1971 David Bowie was almost a hasbeen. In 1969, in the wake of the moon landing he'd had an enormous worldwide hit with *Space Oddity*, but his subsequent singles had been far from successful, and his albums were gradually pushing him underground. Ziggy Stardust made him a megastar almost overnight. In hindsight the creation of Ziggy Stardust seems unduly calculated, but at the time his success seemed entirely natural – a spokesman for a generation which was about to find itself embroiled in glam rock. Ziggy Stardust was a bi-sexual beat Messiah, a flame-haired yob in lipgloss and mascara, silver jumpsuit and platform boots – a strange hybrid of the androgynous spaceman, the rent-boy Elvis and rock'n'roll glitter queen. Bowie said, 'I wasn't at all surprised "Ziggy Stardust" made my career. I packaged a totally credible plastic rock star – much better than any sort of Monkees fabrication. My plastic rocker was much more plastic than anybody's.'

Clothes, though vital to the success of Ziggy, were nothing compared to the influence of the haircut. For the cover of the *Ziggy Stardust* LP Bowie's hair had been cut into a blonde crop, and though it was a complete change from the long locks seen on the Garboesque cover of *Hunky Dory* (his previous LP), it was not the definitive Ziggy. This was cut by Suzy Fussey in February 1972. Suzy worked at the Evelyn Paget hair salon in Beckenham, South London, close to where Bowie and his wife Angie lived at a place called Haddon Hall. Angie's hair had already been cut by Suzy (and subsequently dyed red, white and blue) when Angie asked her to come to Haddon Hall to work on David's.

Between the three of them they fashioned the Ziggy Stardust haircut, using some recent copies of French and German *Vogue*, a potent German dye called Red Hot Red, liberal amounts of peroxide and a formidable setting lotion called Guard (actually a dandruff treatment). After two days of trial and error, Suzy Fussey's Ziggy Stardust haircut was born: a scarlet rooster cut with a blow-dried puff-ball front and a razored back. (When Bowie's manager Tony Defries first saw Ziggy's hair he reputedly dreamt up a scheme for marketing Ziggy Stardust dolls with day-glo hair, which sang 'Wham! Bam! Thank you, ma'am!' But these were never actually made.) Bowie was so happy with the outcome that he later engaged Fussey as the Spiders' full time personal hairdresser.

The Ziggy haircut epitomized the androgyny of glam rock and, copied by both boys and girls (it was as easy for either sex), became the hit of 1973. Not only was the Ziggy Stardust persona influential during the heady days of that year, but throughout the late seventies and early eighties the image of the day-glo rock'n'roll messiah was used and abused by countless pop stars, including Toyah, Richard Butler (The Psychedelic Furs), Siouxsie Sioux, Gary Numan, Steve Strange, John Foxx (Ultravox) and Peter Murphy (Bauhaus), who even covered the song *Ziggy Stardust* with surprising chart success in the early eighties.

The 'Ziggy Stardust' concept – with the glamour shock tactics and three-minute blitzkrieg pop songs – is one of the most important (and most enduring) aspects of British youth culture, emerging in a time of musical indulgence, sartorial apathy and increasing American cultural imperialism, while predating punk rock by four years.

Even though Ziggy Stardust was a self-confessed 'plastic' pop star, next to him the others looked like they were made out of wood.

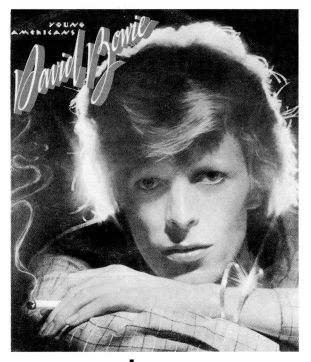

young american

On the sleeve of his *Young Americans* LP (1975), David Bowie finally bid his glam rock days goodbye, while brazenly seeking the attentions of the rapidly expanding soul market. He had his new record – a lovely collection of cod-soul, recorded at Sigma Sound Studio in Philadelphia and Electric Ladyland in New York, with the help of a positively funky John Lennon and a then unknown Luther Vandross – and he had his new haircut, one which again was copied the world over.

ziggy stardust

David Bowie's *Aladdin Sane* LP sleeve (RCA Records, 1973). The second iconographic version of the Ziggy Stardust hairdo. The stripe across Bowie's face was apparently inspired by the lightning flash design on a ring once worn by Elvis, and then copied from the National Panasonic logo.

Bowie's *Pin Ups* LP sleeve (RCA Records, 1973). The androgynous beast leaning on Bowie's shoulder was Twiggy, the perfect compliment to Bowie's shell-shocked Ziggy. The false masks were copied by every nascent glam rocker in town.

Bowie's *Diamond Dogs* LP sleeve (RCA Records, 1974) with the painting by Guy Peellaert. After the publication of *Rock Dreams*, his book of rock 'n' roll airbrushed paintings (captioned by Nik Cohn), Peellaert was much in demand. Bowie was the first person to use him for an LP sleeve (the Rolling Stones were next, with *It's Only Rock 'n' Roll*), depicting him here as half man, half beast . . . from androgyny to 'andogyny'.

bryan ferry

the shag

The rooster cut, or shag, defined the look of seventies man on both sides of the Atlantic. The sexual ambivalence which had surrounded long hair in the late sixties had wounded the considerable male ego, one which was far happier ensconced in something shorter, sexier, and far more rugged. It was essentially a dishevelled and unruly mane with short spiky tufts on top and shoulder-length strands down the back. A descendant of mod, first popularized by Rod Stewart who, throughout the whole flower-power era, retained a cocky Jack-the-lad demeanour, as well as his mod brush.

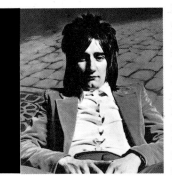

When Bryan Ferry came down to live in London in 1970, he was, fortuitously, introduced to both fashion designer Anthony Price and hairdresser Keith Wainwright in the same evening, at the same party, by a mutual friend called Juliet (later Ferry's girlfriend). With an eye to the grand design for Roxy Music, he engaged these two exponents of urban chic, asking Price to make and design his clothes, and Keith (he was always just Keith) to cut his hair.

Keith owned Smile, Britain's first unisex salon, and it was here that he first cut Ferry's hair. The braying crooner first asked to have his hair dyed jet black. 'This was unheard of at the time,' remembers Keith. 'It was the late hippy period when everyone wanted fresh, clean, healthy, natural looking hair. And in comes Bryan Ferry demanding to be dyed.'

Ferry originally sported a 'Budgie' hairstyle as worn by Adam Faith (another of Smile's clients) in the TV series of the same name, but between them Anthony Price and Keith came up with a far more suitable long dark quiff. Smile was the first salon in the country to champion dyed hair, with obvious effect on the gatefold sleeve of Roxy's second LP, *For Your Pleasure*, giving saxophonist Andy Mackay a green space-age D.A. 'Hair colouring was quite new at the time,' says Keith, 'and when the LP came out we were inundated with people wanting Andy's and Bryan's haircuts. They were the only two in the group who really cared about the way they looked.'

hair by keith

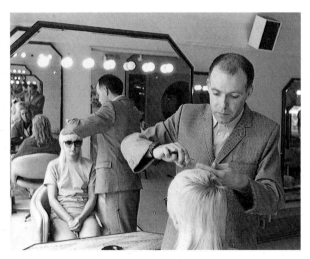

Keith Wainwright's career has traversed all the fads and fancies of the past twenty years. In 1969 he opened Europe's first unisex hair salon, Smile; in the early seventies he introduced the idea of coloured hair for men, pre-empting punk in the process; in the eighties he played a large part in the haircut revolution which evolved from the new romantics. One of the most influential hairdressers of postwar Britain, Bermondsey-born Keith (now in his forties) continues to innovate where others just imitate.

'these foolish things'

For Ferry's first solo record, *These Foolish Things*, Keith gave him the ultimate Roxy icon. 'The cover of *These Foolish Things* is just one big combing job. His hair is actually quite long and tucked around the side and back, because he wouldn't have it cut. This haircut was probably more popular than any other I've ever done. But the haircut I used to give people who wanted one was nothing like the one Ferry had himself, it was something quite different. They would have been really disappointed if I'd given them the real thing.' In 1973 rock stars just didn't look like this.

re-make/re-model

In 1970 a twenty-five-year-old New-
castle art student decided to
change the course of popular
music. He put together a futuristic
rock band called Roxy Music, a pop
art ensemble which bridged the
gap between the heavily defined
areas of rock (the LP market) and
pop (most definitely the singles
market) with a sophisticated yet
outlandish music, a blend of nos-
talgic cinematic glamour, Pop Art,
insinuated sex and tarty, lascivious
stage outfits.

The future that Bryan Ferry
painted was highly desirable, and
Roxy Music's 45s (*Virginia Plain*,
Pyjamarama, *Street Life* etc.) and
33s (*Roxy Music*, *For Your Pleasure*, *Stranded* etc.) sold well in all
parts of the world – apart from,
ironically enough, considering the
visual territory Ferry had plun-
dered, America, where the band's
camp projections were completely
alien to an audience used to James
Taylor, Crosby Stills Nash & Young,
Carole King and Chicago. In 1972
rock stars just didn't look like this.

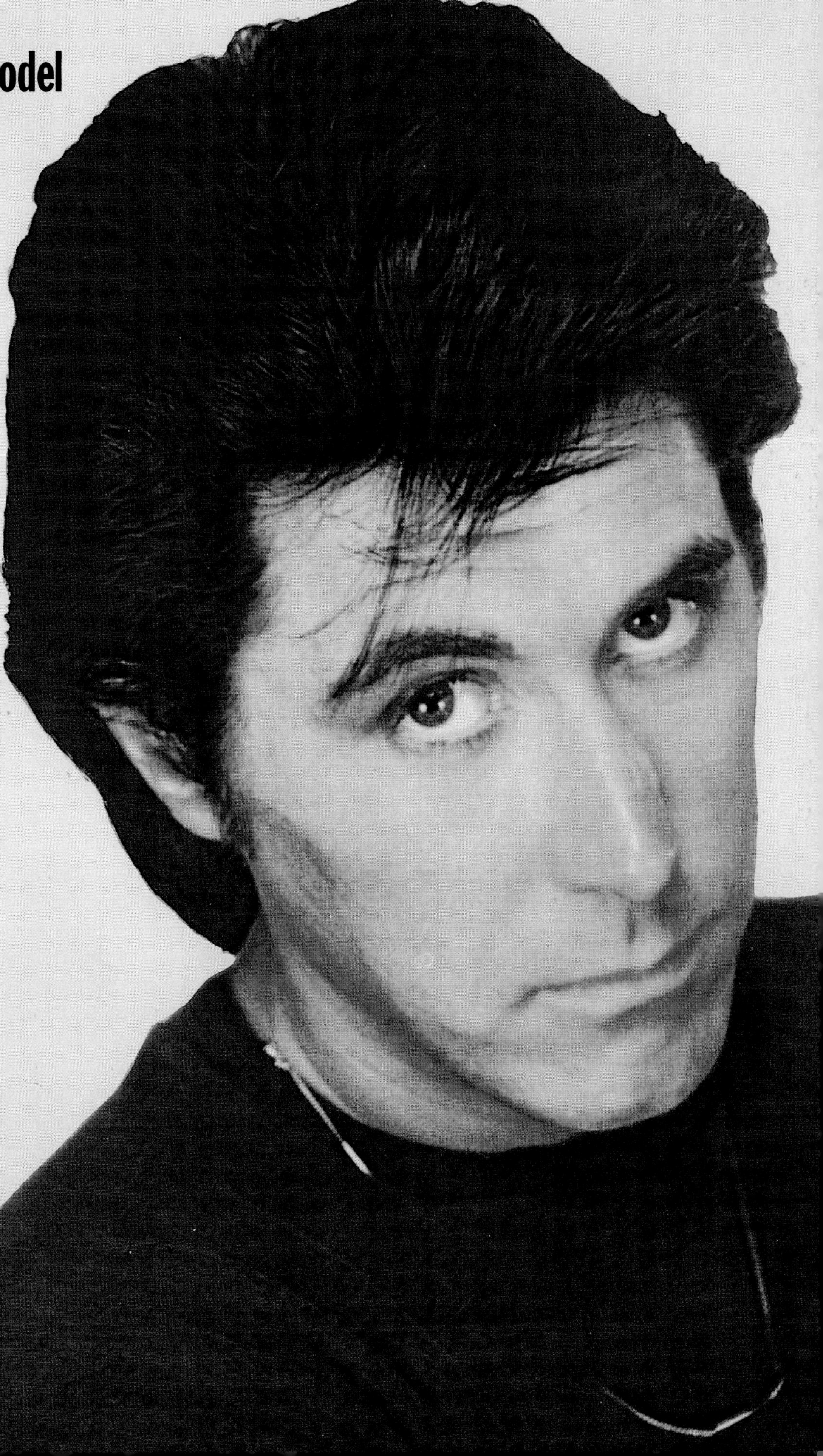

Bryan Ferry
on the cover of
These Foolish Things,
1973. Really inimitable.

skinheads

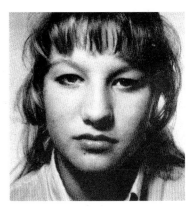

While black America was fashioning a haircult out of racial and political hope and idealism, the Afro, a style of hair and attitude was emerging amongst the British working class young which was far from idealistic – the skinhead. First emerging during 1968, these juvenile rednecks who hated long hair, sub-cultural deviancy, anything in fact remotely bourgeois, constituted a powerful working-class reaction to middle-class hippiedom and self-satisfaction.

Skinheads came initially from the rougher parts of London; malcontents from local authority council housing and tower blocks, they became the most violent British youth cult ever, engaging in gang warfare at the grounds of the English football teams they supported: Tottenham, Chelsea and West Ham.

Their look was a caricature of uncompromising, working-class strength: tight short trousers (Sta-Prest pants or bleached Levi's), big boots (the brown, eight eyelet Air Wear, the British Army two-piece NCB: 'boots like dodgem cars', noted Nik Cohn), button-down Ben Sherman shirts, Brutus and Jaytex shirts and braces; but most expressive of all was the crop – a severe anti-fashion cut which presented the meanest of faces to the world.

Mods had often worn their hair less than half an inch long, but skinheads turned cropped heads into a uniform. At first they were called many things (by themselves as well as other people): 'peanuts', 'lemons',

'skulls', 'cropheads' or 'boiled eggs', but it was the more aggressive 'skinhead' which stuck. Though there was never any rule as to how the hair should fall at the back of the head (it either sank into your collar, or ended in a 'Boston' or a sharp curve), there were strict guidelines about its length. Hair was cut with an electric razor, set to one of four lengths (in extreme cases, when a longer cut was required, five).

Obviously the shorter haircuts were most menacing, and hard cases prided themselves with their 'Number Ones'. Some skinheads sported mutton-chop sideburns, an aberration picked up by Jesse Hector's punk band The Gorillas. Skinhead girls in the late sixties and early seventies almost always wore the feather cut – cropped on top with wisps of hair falling over the face, ears and neck.

Skinheads were in decline until the birth of punk, when they reappeared in even greater numbers; their affiliations, though, with the punk movement were always ambivalent, with a distressingly large percentage of the 'new' skinheads involving themselves with fascist political movements.

In the eighties the skinhead has largely disappeared again, his only real legacy being his hair, which lives on atop art students, neurotic boy outsiders, graphic designers and painters the world over. There has been a revolt into style; a skinhead haircut still means *alternative*, though the implications are no longer violent. They're artistic.

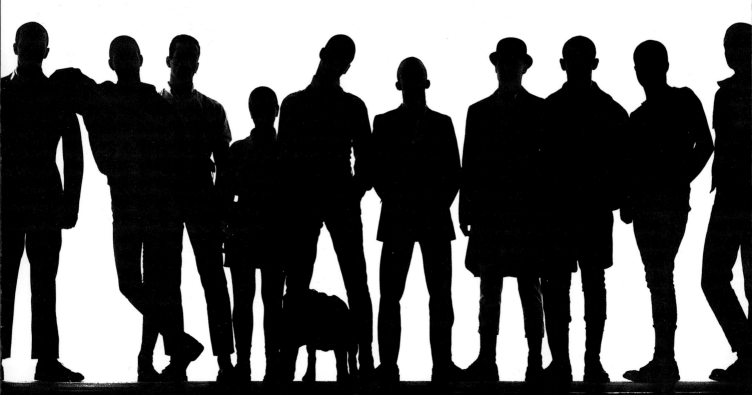

Skinhead by Richard Allen (1970); the skinheads and their haircuts were eulogized in several pulp paperbacks by exploitation writer Richard Allen in the early seventies. *Skinhead* was published in 1971, a piece of subculture literature which was aimed at schoolkids old enough to have heard of the 'cropped-haired thugs' and young and impressionable enough to believe the ridiculous escapades of the proto-skinhead Joe Hawkins. *Skinhead* was an immediate hit and the publishers, realizing they had a substantial success on their hands, responded with seventeen more Richard Allen titles, of which ten were skinhead related: *Suedehead* (1971), *Skinhead Escapes* (1972), *Skinhead Girls* (1972), *Trouble For Skinhead* (1973), *Sorts* (1971), *Top Gear Skin* (1974), *Skinhead Farewell* (1974), *Terrace Terrors* (1974), *Dragon Skins* (1975) and *Knuckle Girls* (1977).

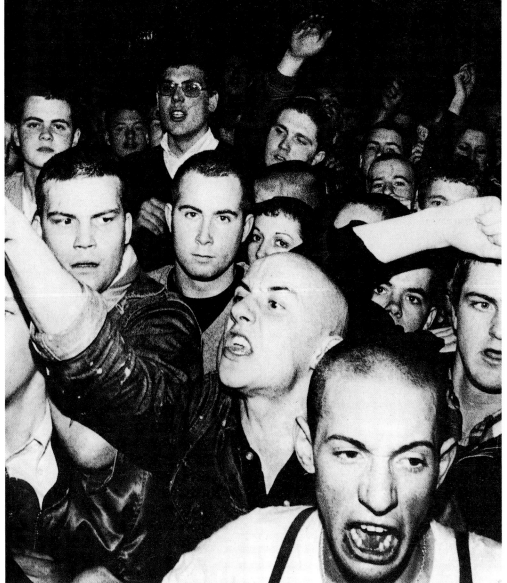

A skinhead crowd pledges its allegiance.

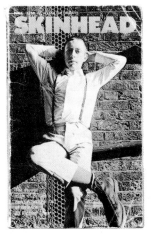

Allen's books are mostly lurid accounts of gratuitous sex and violence, with a collective subtext which almost always seems to condone both racism and sexism. As pulp fiction goes, this is some of the most extreme, and some of the worst written; though, almost inevitably, first editions of the early books are now quite valuable.

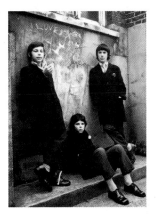

Suedehead by Richard Allen (1971); although some of Allen's youth groups were the result of a vivid (if infertile) imagination, suedeheads actually existed. Though their clothes were marginally different from those worn by skinheads – car coats and donkey jackets, scruffy mods with umbrellas – the suedehead hair was precisely that: a grown-out crop, sometimes worn with furry sideburns.

The menacing symmetry of a gang of perfectly outfitted skinheads.

disco!

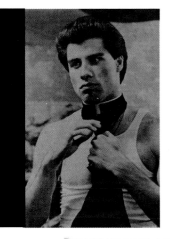

Saturday Night Fever (1977) was one of the highest grossing and most influential movies of the whole 'Me Decade', putting disco firmly on the map and taking it out of the clubs and into the charts. John Travolta also became a star through this movie, although his blow-dried hair proved less influential than the Bee Gees' homogenized dance soundtrack. Travolta plays a one-dimensional Italian hardware store assistant from Brooklyn called Tony Manero, whose sole pleasure in life is dancing. In the film Manero becomes a disco demigod, and though Travolta achieved rather similar fame in real life, his thatch never achieved the notoriety of the one worn by that other famous 'Italian', Tony Curtis.

farrah

By 1976, as the tousled blonde beauty of the American television programme *Charlie's Angels*, Farrah Fawcett had become the world's number one pin-up. The mildly erotic posters of her were some of the best-selling of the decade and though her co-stars in the programme, Jaclyn Smith and Kate Jackson, achieved stardom too, it was Farrah, with her mass of golden locks, whom the public took to their hearts. Not surprisingly, Fawcett soon felt typecast, and left the series after only one season (it continued to run until 1981), to seek out more serious roles. She has received favourable reviews for some of her work in the late seventies and early eighties, but she seems forever trapped by her proto-bimbo image as the Angel with the flowing mane and eager smile.

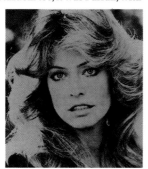

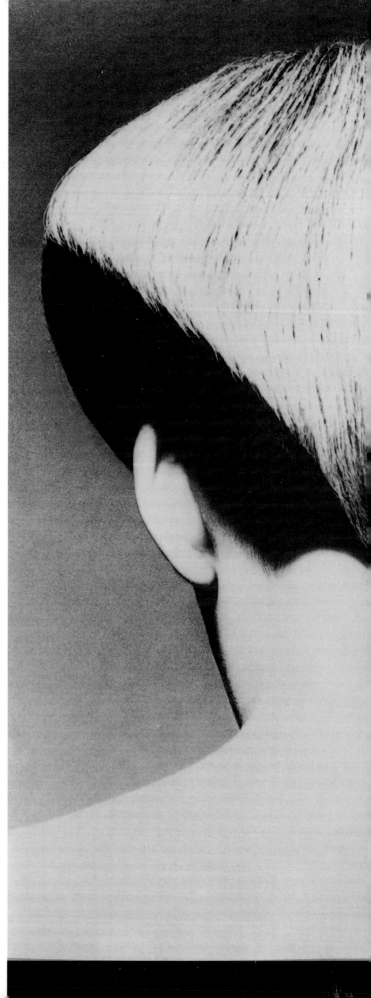

the wedge

the soul underground

The wedge was invented by Trevor Sorbie, a hairdresser at one of Vidal Sassoon's London salons, in 1974. Originally created specifically for girls, it was quickly devoured by their boyfriends, who flaunted their newly acquired aerodynamic masterpieces in nightclubs from Ilford to Southend (along the A13, the backbone of British club culture). Adopted by the soul fraternity as a tonsorial flag, the wedge was not only a precursor to a decade of soul boy culture, it also became its most durable metaphor.

Quite unlike all those 'rock culture' haircuts (long, lank, and dirty), the wedge was, to quote Peter York, 'the uniform for the southern English, club-going, working-class soul stylist.' As pop archivists are always keen to point out, the mid seventies were clearly polarized, and in the cathedrals of dance along the A13, the wedge-wearing funkateers enjoyed the euphonious delights of imported American soul music – third generation r&b and progressive pomp rock just didn't get a look in. On the southern soul scene the clothes you wore were as important as the steps you traced on the dance floor; but neither was as important as your wedge.

York described its construction in detail: 'When they first cut it and blow it dry they keep on brushing the sides flat, pushing them back underneath the long bits at the crown so the bob part of it is resting on the pushed-back horizontal part. The stylists' trick then is to *let it go*, so it springs out, the long bits bouncing out on top of the side, all that bouncing volume disappearing into razored flatness with nothing hippy or impromptu around the neck.' In 'All You Have To Do Is Win', an article published in *The Face* in May 1985 concerning the ubiquity of soul boy culture in the eighties, Robert Elms describes seeing his first real 'soul boy' on a London District Line underground train about 1975. This creature's clothes were shocking, the very antithesis of seventies excess '. . . but it was his hair that really got you; it was both long and short at the same time, heavy on top and falling over one eye, but karate-chop short at the neck. It was like a lop-sided pudding-basin but streaked as if this boy had spent time in the sun.'

The soul movement was one which body-swerved punk, re-emerging two years later in a dingy London nightclub called Billy's just in time for the beginning of what became labelled the 'style' decade. Unlike the punk haircut, which was immediately recognized as a totem of rebellious style culture, the wedge was not acknowledged a socio-cultural influence until the eighties.

The original wedge, cut by Trevor Sorbie at Vidal Sassoon, 1974.

heavy metal contradictions

mad axeman!

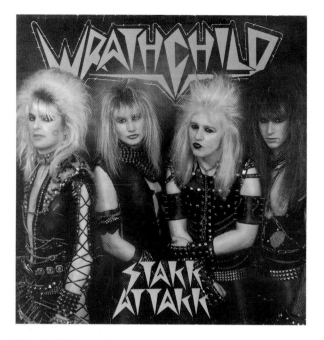

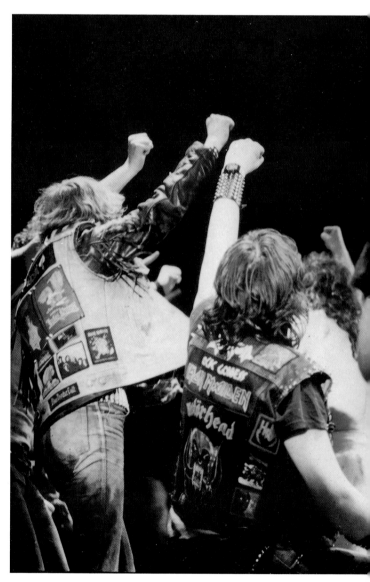

Wrath Child, seen here on the cover of their 1984 LP *Stakk Attakk*, are typical of a certain kind of airbrushed heavy metal in the eighties, the supposed macho men of slick modern HM appear as a gang of renegade hair dressers. In 1987 *i-D* magazine called this phenomenon 'Elnett Rock': 'Sunset Boulevard's clubs play host to a metal subcult which owes more to Max Factor than Muddy Waters, and a night-time cruise along Sunset Strip will reveal hundreds of pristinely presented metal mutants who make Boy George and "Purple Rain" period Prince look underdressed.'

Today there are massive contradictions in the way heavy metal rock stars present themselves. There is also much inhouse bickering between the many different HM factions – between the greboes and the Satanists and the HM Christians, between the exponents of thrash metal, speed metal, or plain old heavy metal. Some, like Wrath Child, mix studs'n'leather with lipstick and hairspray; some, like Iron Maiden, just come across as beery lads; and others manage to combine the two.

But forgetting the way in which, over the years, the codes have become confused, and ignoring each band's chosen idiosyncracies, two things remain the same: everything still centres around the perpetuation of guitar as phallic symbol; and all the groups invariably sound the same.

the clone zone

The boys own club

In 1972 the gay male fraternities in the villages of New York City and San Francisco started their own small army, a narcissistic subcult which began apeing traditionally masculine dress, and thereby initiating a very special kind of style warfare. By fusing various elements of male costume, and scrambling the typical codes of machismo, they not only undermined and ultimately diffused these images of rampant heterosexuality but created new composite gay images.

A prerequisite for joining these new battalions of style was the closely cropped hair, a severe head-dress totally at odds with established images of gay men. This haircut was an illusion of irony, as the appropriated G.I. crop soon became synonymous with gay culture.

Later in the decade, these new corporate images of homosexuality would be popularized by the butch disco squad, The Village People (cop, construction worker, biker, cowboy, etc.), but the look which most successfully permeated the mainstream was the lumberjack or woodsman: the tight blue jeans, field boots, plaid shirt, and close cropped G.I. style hair.

Of course, this look, along with all the others, soon became saddled with the by now familiar gigantic handlebar moustache, the one completely uncompromising tool of modern gay symbolism.

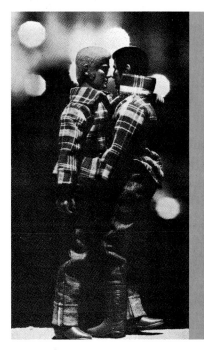

headbanger

Here we see the unkempt hair of an obsessed heavy metal 'headbanger'; often carrying cardboard guitars to concerts and clubs, the headbangers would ape their heroes (hard rock groups like Motorhead, Status Quo, Lynyrd Skynyrd) in dress, style of hair and the way they played their monotonous bass-leaden boogie (often note-for-repetitive-note). They originated in the early seventies, though are still commonplace today, as is their unshapely, unwashed and characterless long hair.

Confrontation: with her geometric war-paint, technicolour mop and hollow eyes, *Sex* shop assistant Jordan was a sight to make regular folks' hair stand on end.

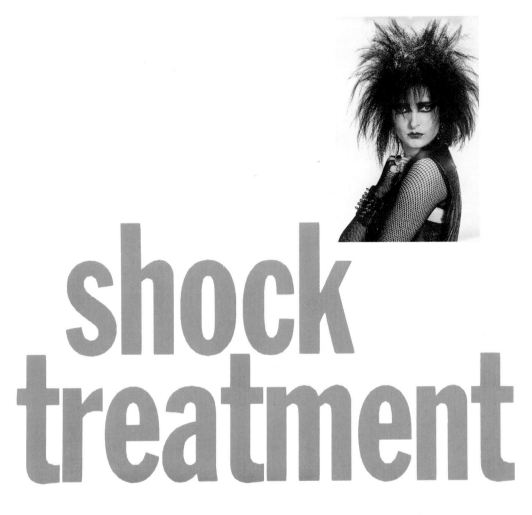

shock treatment

In 1976 punk said goodbye to all that. Anarchy, insurrection and short spiky hair replaced the excesses of the early seventies. And as punk was a nihilistic movement, it adopted a nihilistic haircut, albeit one invented by an American singer called Richard·Hell in 1974.

What followed was the biggest cultural upheaval since the fifties, a glorious celebration of youth which almost succeeded in ignoring its subcultural origins. Welcome to the blank generation . . .

mohawk

There is still much confusion over just what a 'Mohican' or 'Mohawk' haircut actually is. The Mohawks were an Indian tribe from Iroquois in New York State, while the Mohicans (Mohegans) were from Connecticut. The word Mohican seems to have evolved as a generic term for the high Indian head-dress through poor journalism and television. The head-dress, a variation on the Trojan plume, was actually worn by the Huron ('bristle-head' in French), Omaha and Osage tribes, who cut and shaved their children's hair from an early age in many different styules, one of which, the Mohican (meaning 'wolf'), was a long thin cut representing a line of buffaloes outlined against the horizon at sunset.

For nearly all North American Indians hair not only symbolized the relationship between themselves and their natural surroundings, but the strange relationship between the Indian and his spirit. Consequently hair became emblematic in many ways, not least in the field of battle. The Indians wore their Mohican haircuts as acts of defiance, daring the enemy into attacking them, trying to take their scalp in the process. According to Chris Wroblewski and Nelly Gommez-Vaez's book *City Tribes* (1984), the Osage and Ohama tribes used to stiffen their locks with bear grease or walnut oil, so the hair would resemble the horn of a bull, and thus appear more frightening still.

The Mohican hairstyle was picked up by both American rockabillies and British Teddy boys at the beginning of the fifties (perhaps through an early television series about Canadian Indians), though their 'Apache' haircuts usually consisted of a flat oblong slab in the middle of the scalp, with the sides of the head shaven. (It is likely that Elvis Presley himself sported a Mohawk during the summer of 1950, and jazzman Sonny Rollins is reputed to have worn a Mohawk haircut during the early sixties.)

The Mohican only really came into its own as a totemic youth hairstyle in 1977, with the consolidation of punk rock in Britain. By the end of that year, the Mohican had replaced ordinary spiky haircuts as the most extreme example of the new pop culture. A punk haircut was relatively easy to revert, but the colossal Mohawk head-dress was impossible to disguise, consequently becoming the strongest visual symbol of punk's radical posture.

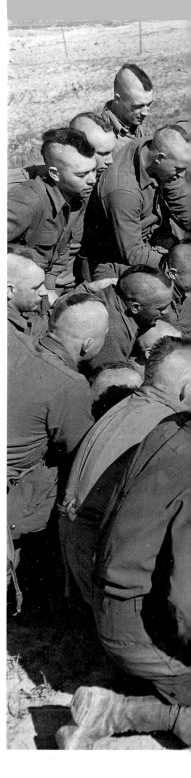

taxi driver

Robert de Niro as Travis Bickle, the cabbie in Martin Scorsese's 1976 film *Taxi Driver*. Bickle is an ex-Marine who turns to taxi driving to help relieve his insomnia. Prowling the sleazy streets of New York at night he is disgusted by the crime and filth around him. He decides to turn himself into Manhattan's social con-science in the guise of a catch-all vigilante, but not before he shaves his head into a replica of a Mohawk headdress.

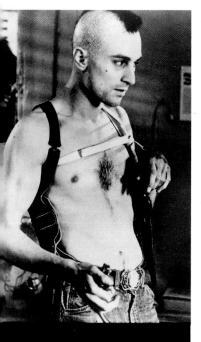

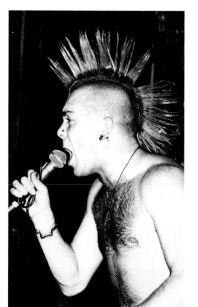

Watty of The Exploited, a noisy post-punk band, sporting his own interpretation of the Mohawk.

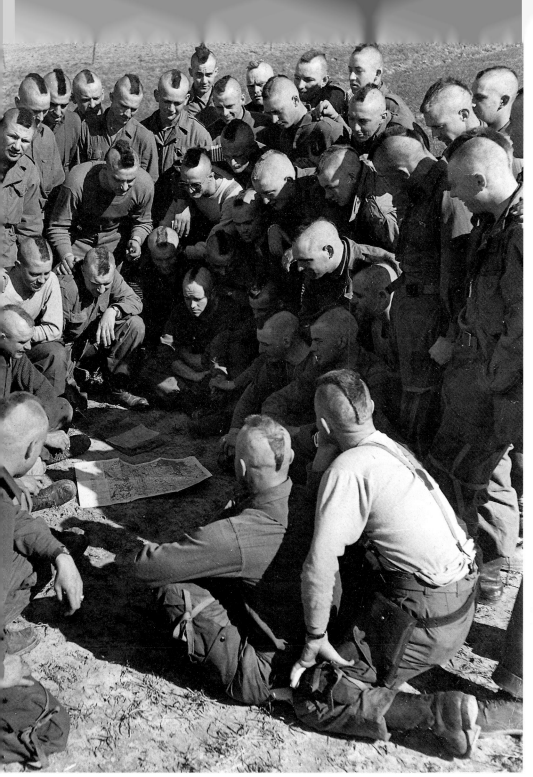

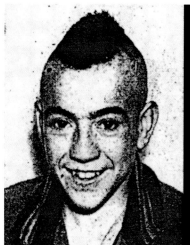

the first punk in town

Mancunian hairdresser George Mason was, so he thought, a master of publicity. Twice during 1951 he devised PR schemes intended to have Manchester's young men flocking to his tiny Wythenshawe hair salon. The first gimmick involved the construction of a barbershop atop a motorized lorry which toured Wythenshawe during a local pageant, with Mr Mason attending to his customers as it went. The second was considerably more successful: Mason advertised a gift of £1 to be given to the first boy to turn up at his salon and ask for a 'Mohican'.

The winner was a small fifteen-year-old errand boy called John Ross from nearby Woodhouse Park, and for his pound he was expected to tell inquirers where he got such a 'savage' hairstyle and to recommend a visit (for something less exciting, but equally striking). Greater Manchester wasn't exactly struck by the Mohican idea, though it certainly remembered Mr. Mason's name, and he even earned himself a write-up in *Hairdressers' Journal*. As for little John Ross, one wonders how he would have reacted if he had known that he was twenty-five years ahead of his time.

Arras, France, 23 March 1945. U.S. paratroopers, their hair cut Mohawk style for luck and *esprit de corps*, are briefed for the next day's jump across the Rhine. This is the first available photograph of anyone using the 'Mohican' style of hairstyle since the Indian tribes themselves.

esprit de corps

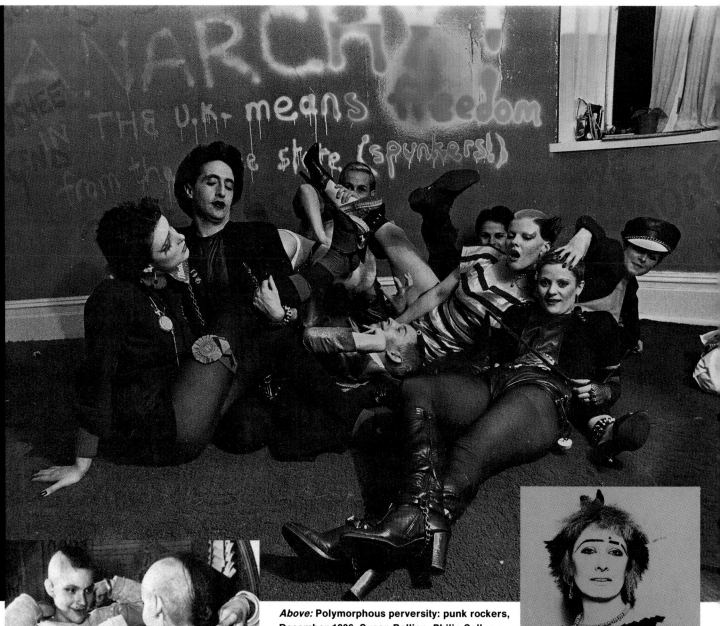

Above: Polymorphous perversity: punk rockers, December 1986. Susan Ballion, Philip Sallon, Sue Catwoman, Steve Havoc and other members of the Bromley Contingent.

An AP Wire-photo from 1951: 'Los Angeles, June 26 – TEENAGE GIRL JOINS RANKS OF BRAVES – Mohican haircuts, which have recently become the fad among young boys, spread into the feminine ranks today, Josephine Amaya, 17, combs out the pig-tailed stubble which she adopted with the aid of her 14-year-old sister, Velia, sitting in as barber. As a concession to femininity she left a pig-tail dangling down her back.'

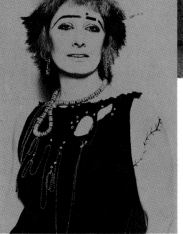

Above: Zandra Rhodes was the first fashion designer to jump on the punk bandwagon, creating a range of ripped and torn haute couture clothes covered in safety pins.

proto-punks

Below: Sid Vicious pictured in early punk fanzine *Scum*. Easily the most copied of all male punk haircuts. *Left:* Alienation. Seminal punk icon Sue Catwoman – short, dyed scalp, black feline spikes and pronounced eye make-up, Catwoman's severe image was one of the most photographed during punk's heyday, though it defied imitation. (It was itself a multicoloured copy of the 1950 Banana Shingle cut . . . like a Mephistopheles wig.)

Johnny Rotten (John Lydon) perhaps personified everything vital about the punk movement. He was outspoken, uncompromising, at turns both intensely animated and obstinately lethargic, and he was a complete individual. Sid Vicious might have had the total punk look, but Rotten had the attitude.

In 1974, though, things were different, as Rotten used to hang around Hawkwind, a band of psychedelic hippy degenerates. During the early days of punk Lydon became notorious for wearing a torn and customized t-shirt which read 'I Hate Pink Floyd', though in 1974 he was one of their most ardent fans. He had long red hair (he dyed it with henna), wore a greatcoat and advocated listening to Roy Harper.

Around the same time Malcolm McLaren, the manager of the New York Dolls, was trying to put together an anarchic supergroup, which eventually became the Sex Pistols. He searched for two years for the right members, trying to recruit both Richard Hell (then the driving force in the New York art band Television) and New York Doll Johnny Thunders, before finding Steve Jones, Paul Cook, Glen Matlock and eventually John Lydon. McLaren not only wanted Hell because he had incredible stage presence and an unnerving, seering voice, but also because he had great hair.

In the autumn of 1974 celebrity photographer Robert Mapplethorpe took the first arty picture of Television, in which Richard Hell sported his freshly customized haircut – he had taken a pair of scissors to his thatch and cut it in short clumps of varying lengths which made him end up looking like a dog who'd just been through a carwash. This photograph was published in Andy Warhol's *Interview* at the end of the year, and was seen by McLaren, then in New York. On returning to London he put the picture of Hell up on the wall in Sex, the shop he ran with Vivienne Westwood in the King's Road.

Lydon, now a frequent visitor to the shop, saw the picture and promptly cut his hair in the same fashion. This would have been in early 1975, proving once and for all that what became known around the world as a British style revolution was actually stolen from America, from Richard Hell, the original punk. Lydon was soon spotted by McLaren, and coerced into the Sex Pistols as their lyricist, spokesman and singer, becoming, for the media at least, the world's first, most dangerous punk rocker.

Punk was the haircut which said 'Fuck off', a multi-faceted icon which had the ultimate shock value – the haircut as Abstract Expressionism. There was no ambiguity about these short, sharp, shorn locks – this was 'No

Future, No Quarter'. Haute coiffure this was not. In 1976 long hair was suddenly considered reactionary, the symbol of an older, redundant subculture which had grown fat and pompous in the name of hippiedom. (Such was the immersion of America in 'freak' culture that when the short-haired British punks first toured there in 1977–78 they were called 'faggots' by the young long-haired, pot-bellied rednecks of the Midwest. Oh, how things change!) Punks were out to change everything; their object? – to chase introspection and indulgence from the building, to stop the world and start again, to create havoc and have a good time in the process.

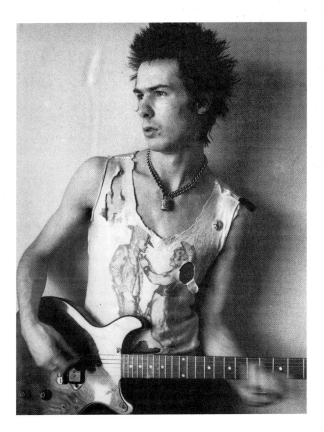

punk

The early punks were a mixture of art students, hippies, soul boys and fashion groupies, and their clothes and haircuts reflected this. But when punk got into its stride, when it went overground, all those new recruits had an awful lot of catching up to do, not least they had to cut their hair and style it in the appropriate 'D.I.Y.' fashion.

But what to use on the fledgling barnet? In the days before hair gel anything and everything came in handy, everything from food colouring, sugar, lard, toothpaste, washing up liquid, margarine and butter to cooking oil, glue, soap, and egg white (favoured by Sid Vicious). Tony James (then of Generation X) says that, in order to obtain the perfect hedgehog, he used a combination of lemon juice, spit and orange juice: 'I used to walk round smelling like a carton of Kia-Ora.' Ultimately punk changed the way people looked, felt, and consumed; it also changed the course of popular music for good. Until the New York Dolls, the Ramones and Television came along, no one in a rock group had seen their feet or their ears since the mid sixties.

It didn't take long for punk to go public, and not only did fashion designer Zandra Rhodes produce a collection based entirely on the punk

'The sickest, seediest step in a rock world that thought it had seen it all' (*The Daily Mail*, December 1986)

'No other subculture illustrates more clearly the importance of theft and transformation in the development of style than punk. It incorporates conscious reference to the legacy of all preceding subcultures.' (Helen Rees)

look in late 1977, but hairdressers across the country began incorporating punk styles into their repertoire, with cuts variously termed 'Pretty Punk' and 'Hedgehog Head'. One of the few hairdressers to be really innovative during this period was Ray Bird, then working at Alan's Hairdressers in the King's Road. He cut leopard-skin markings, words and figures – 'rebel', '999' – and other shock designs, like safety pins and arrows, into his customers' heads; one Sex Pistols fan even asked for his scalp to be adorned with the words 'Sid Vicious – 1957–1979'.

Like everything before it, the effect of punk was quickly diffused, though Billy Idol can still be seen parading his designer punk around the stadiums of North America, dressed in expensive black leathers and a lovingly nurtured blonde spiky top. As for John Lydon, the prince of punks retains his hypnotic presence, his autonomy, though sadly, not his original spiky hair.

By the end of the seventies the Great British Punk was as much of a tourist attraction as the Great British Beefeater. If you wanted to see punks you came to London where, in Sloane Square, you could have your picture taken (at 50p a throw) with amiable young boys and girls dressed in deliberately distressed leather jackets and fantastic haircuts doused in Crazy Colour. The haircuts were far more exaggerated, far more colourful than anything that existed during the punk era, haircuts created entirely for American cameras and Japanese television crews. Punk rockers are the only youth cult to have sold themselves in this way (can you imagine skinheads posing for photographs with Scandinavian tourists?) happy in the knowledge that they have become accepted as yet more examples of Great British Eccentricity.

Punks and palaces are now the predominant postcard images of London, helping turn Britain into one huge, sprawling suburban theme park (Heathrow and Gatwick airports being the turnstiles). 'There's not much to choose,' says Peter York, 'between the Changing of the Guard and the King's Road parade these days. They're both part of our Glorious Heritage.'

london, where else?

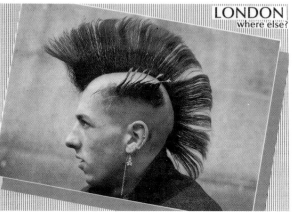

Opposite: The iconic John Lydon, punk's Prince Charming.

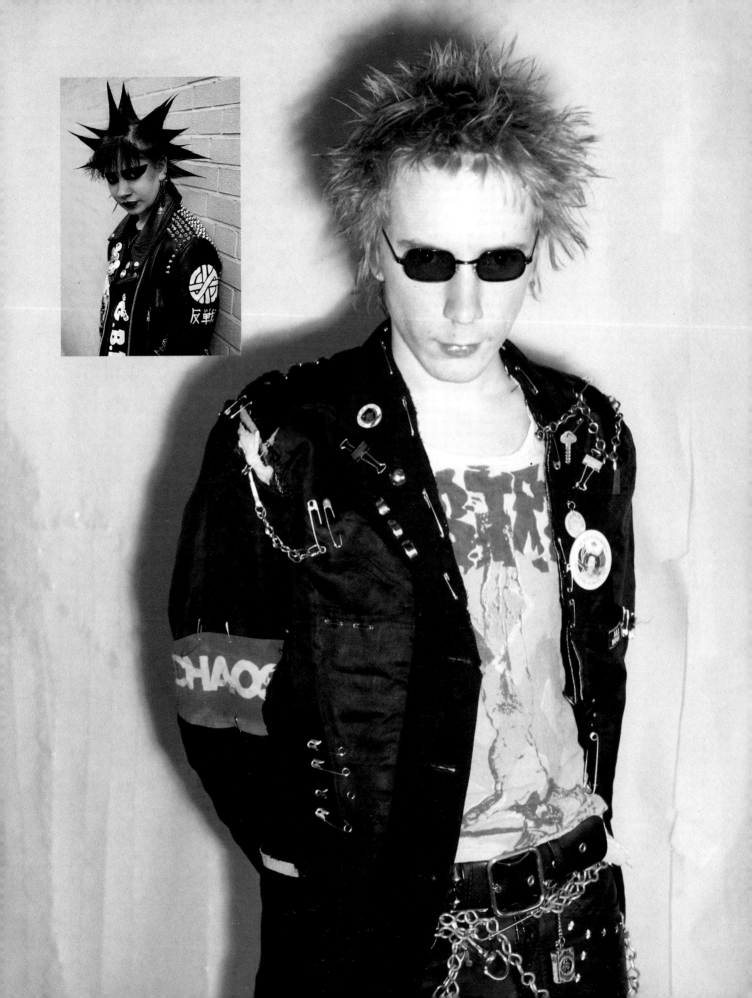

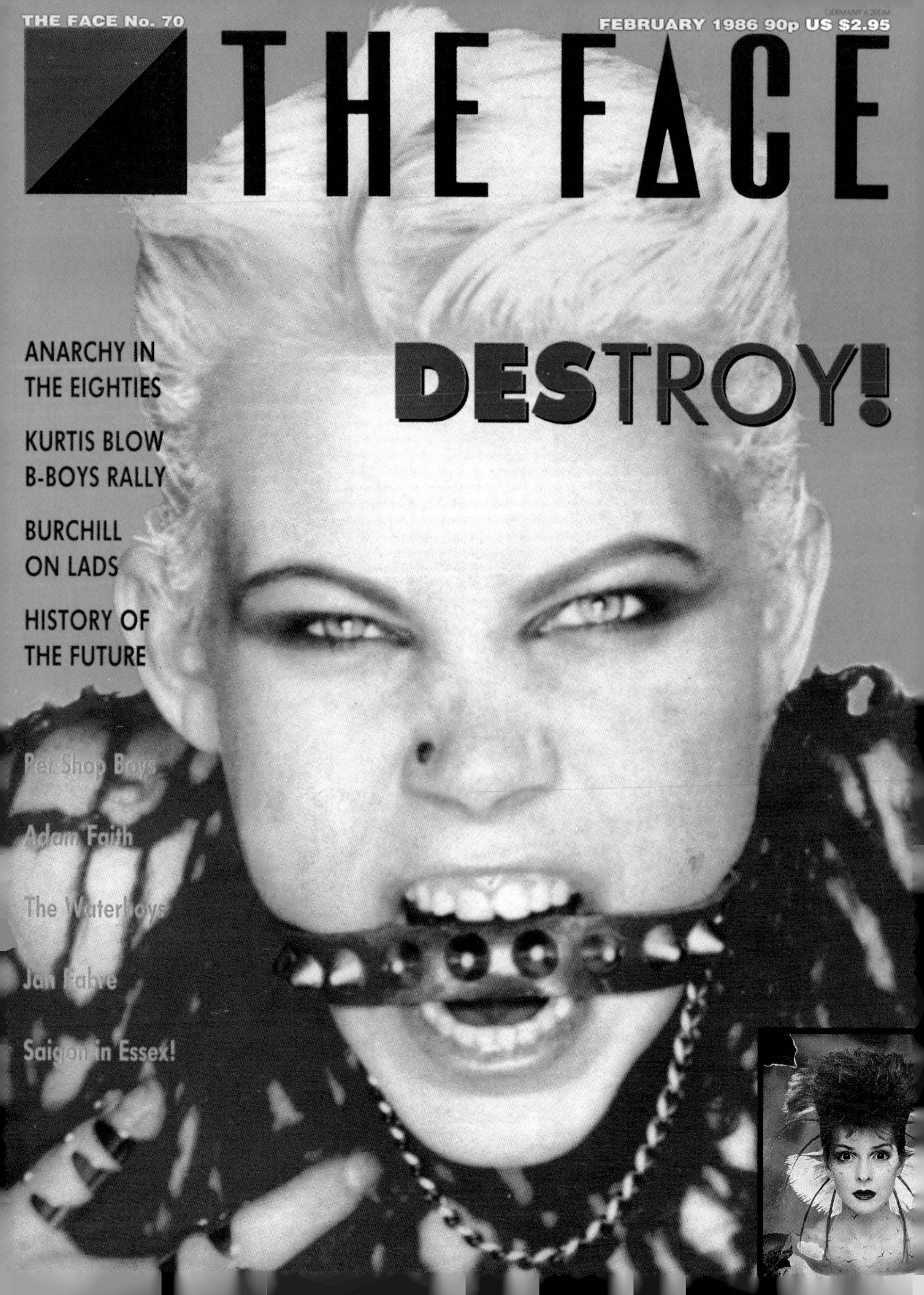

THE FACE No. 70

FEBRUARY 1986 90p US $2.95

GERMANY 6.20DM

THE FACE

DESTROY!

ANARCHY IN
THE EIGHTIES

KURTIS BLOW
B-BOYS RALLY

BURCHILL
ON LADS

HISTORY OF
THE FUTURE

Pet Shop Boys

Adam Faith

The Waterboys

Jan Fabre

Saigon in Essex!

Retro-punk: the ten-year anniversary of punk prompted many celebrations – none better than this brilliant 1986 cover of *The Face*; doubly ironic when you consider that Nick Logan's brainchild was the archetypal magazine of the eighties. Here the hair is styled, gelled, and lovingly art-directed, absolute designer insurrection for absolute beginners.

blonde on blonde

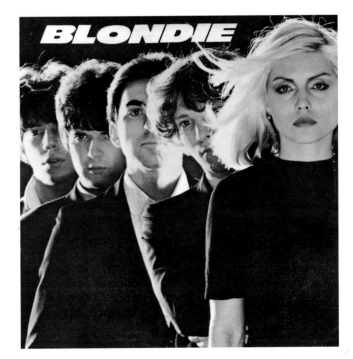

ouch!

Crazy colour, crazy girl! The picture disc of Toyah's 'Brave New World' single (1982); Toyah epitomized plastic, weekend punks, those suburban boys and girls for whom fancy dress was more important than nihilism. Adam Ant would later take the plastic punks into a new era with pop new romanticism, personified by mock anthems like 'Antmusic', 'Kings of the Wild Frontiers', 'Stand and Deliver' and 'Prince Charming'. Toyah's music was as gaudy as her hair, and thankfully just as temporary.

Though Deborah Harry, with her metaphorical appropriation of platinum blonde hair, spray-on micro-skirts and melodic monosyllabic pop became the most acceptable – and ultimately the most successful – of all the punk pin-ups, she never tried to hide the fact that her iconographic hair was dyed; on the record sleeve illustrated here you can even see her brown roots. Blondie's tongue was firmly in its collective cheek. Even their name was a giveaway – a band called Blondie fronted by a girl who obviously dyed her hair. Debbie Harry may have been a sex kitten, but she was certainly no bimbo, and set about exploiting her sexuality before anyone else got a chance.

From the beginnings of the group, Harry was always toying with the ambiguity of pop iconography and the implications of sexual role playing. The endless Monroe comparisons were taken with liberal pinches of salt by both Harry and her boyfriend, band member Chris Stein. The irony was eclipsed when Blondie went on to become one of the most successful pop bands of the late seventies – the supreme global wet dream (they were also one of the first groups to successfully fuse disco and punk).

siouxsie sioux

'tarantula on stilts'

Siouxsie Sioux hasn't seen her real hair since she was sixteen. 'I catch glimpses of it every now and then', she says, 'and I've seen the odd grey hair, but I really don't know what colour my real hair is now. I've kept it dyed since before punk.'

As a schoolgirl in Chislehurst, Kent, Susan X was a determined loner, a reclusive Roxy freak with hair 'down to my bum'. Without a peer group ('I used to like Roxy Music and Bowie, but I never wanted to emulate them like other people') and feeling alienated from her surroundings, she began making day-trips to London, visiting Biba, the King's Road, soaking up the urbanity much like another proto-punk, Paul Weller (who used to come up to London and record the traffic). Gradually she became embroiled in what became known as the Bromley Contingent – cutting her hair into strange shapes and dyeing it funny colours, shopping at jumble sales, wearing outlandish make-up and generally running riot. 'It was a form of rebellion I suppose. I was never happy at school, really miserable, hated it. I was very lonely, but mainly out of choice. As soon as I left I cut my hair … that's when I began to meet different kinds of people. You have to pay for your independence. When I was at school my mum bought all my clothes, so I could never get involved in what was fashionable . . . but then I wouldn't

the hair which spawned a million goths

have wanted to. Leaving was the first chance I had to strike out on my own. I got a strange, perverse thrill from looking the way I did – it was like having a massive surge of adrenalin.

Having met other like-minded punks in London, she, with the Bromley Contingent, began going to gigs and hanging out with the Sex Pistols. In September 1976, at the 100 Club Punk Festival an adhoc Siouxsie and the Banshees (including Sid Vicious) made their first live appearance, stumbling and wailing their way through a twenty-minute rendition of 'The Lord's Prayer'. Flushed with this success Siouxsie decided to form a band proper, and thus started what is now the longest lasting punk band.

Throughout this first period of punk activity Siouxsie's hair was rather typical, a short, sharp shock which was either peroxide or jet black. When the press turned their attention to this outburst of youth-anasia, Siouxsie stepped back: 'The worst thing about the whole punk thing was that people were able to call you something on the street. Being caught out spoiled all the fun'.

It was now that Siouxsie got to grips with the way she looked, dressing in unlikely punk garb, creating her iconographic face mask and cutting her hair into jagged edges. She cut her own hair until 1980 when she enlisted the help of one Roger Taylor, a hairdresser friend of Banshee guitarist John McGeoch. It was with him that she created what has become one of the most influential haircuts of the eighties, the seminal gothic head-dress which was aped by every noir aspirant from Manhattan to Middlesborough.

What is most peculiar is that the girls and boys (this was gothic androgyny) who copied Siouxsie were emulating her haircut, not expressing devotion to the Banshees. To wear your hair *à la* Siouxsie is to belong to the world of the Cramps and the Birthday Party, Bauhaus and The Batcave (which put the goth back into Gotham), of T. Rex and aluminium skulls and cults which go bang! in the dark.

'I knew I wanted something different, it was just a case of trial and error, really. Someone told me about crimpers, and after using them a few times I realized what you could actually do with them. One day I just started hacking and came up with the idea for the look – I wanted a haircut which was gravity defying. Then Roger came along and we've been doing it together ever since.'

She is pleased by the mass emulation, but feels that more than just create a trendy haircut, she has helped change the way in which women present themselves. 'In the twenties women looked very strong. This was a very bolshy period for them, with their austere bobs and straight up and down lines. Women then looked powerful. I've always tried to be the antithesis of the curvy, tanned, blonde bombshell. I can't do much about the curves, but everything else . . .'

gothic locks

In 1978 Robert Smith started the Cure, a post-punk pop group obsessed with adolescent neuroses and sullen melancholy. Five years after their inception, in the spring of 1982, Smith wholeheartedly adopted the gothic look, taking his hairstyle – his thatch noir – from those nocturnal creatures who frequented The Batcave, listened obsessively to the Cramps and dressed entirely in black. Coincidentally this was about the time that Smith began collaborating with the Banshees, and he became the male counterpart to Siouxsie's iconographic gothic nymph; wearing deliberately smudged lipstick, pasty white make-up and those spidery black tresses, Robert Smith became the epitome of the gothic style. In 1986, when he decided to cut off all his hair, leaving a stubborn brown tuft, MTV broadcast news of the event every 30 minutes for 24 hours.

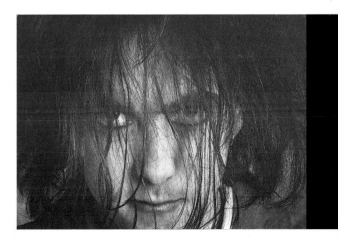

dreadlocks

All the days of the vow of his separation there shall no razor come upon his head: until the days be fulfilled, in that which he separateth himself unto the Lord, he shall be holy, and shall let the locks of the hair of his head grow. (*Numbers* 6:5)

A classic example of dreadlocks worn by a member of a Jamaican Rastafarian sect.

In 1914 Jamaican-born Marcus Garvey founded the Universal Negro Improvement Association, an organization which helped establish a new consciousness among native Jamaicans. Leaving the island in 1916, he set up headquarters in Harlem, New York, rapidly recruiting people to the cause. By 1922 the Association had over seven million members. After spending some time in gaol (convicted of fraud), Garvey was deported and arrived back in Jamaica in 1928, where he involved himself in the politics of black emancipation. In 1929 he prophecied that a black king would soon be crowned in Africa, and that when this happened it would signal the day of redemption for their race. A year later Ras Tafari was crowned Haile Selassie I, Emperor of Ethiopia – Rastafarianism was born. The people had a leader, a spiritual home, and a name.

As the hardcore Rastas began distancing themselves from other Jamaicans, particularly the middle class, they started to evolve their own religious practices, their own code of dress, their own language, a penchant for marajuana (ganga), and the highly distinctive dreadlocks, the real symbol of Rastafarianism. Already an Ethiopian hairstyle, locks were adopted by the Jamaican Rastas in the thirties as an affirmation of their belief (and later re-exported back to Tanzania and Zimbabwe). The name stems from 'fear-locks', because of the fear and dread which they inspire (they are also meant to represent a lion's mane). Uncombed and plaited, the Rastas' hair would fall into flowing locks, extending past the shoulders. Dreadlocks are often portrayed as neat, lovingly nurtured head-dresses, though until recently most Rastas wore their locks in wild styles, (sometimes referred to by Rastas as 'antennae') shooting out at all angles, in great clumps of knotted bush.

Later, after ska and rock steady, reggae music would become the Rastafarian soundtrack, reaching its zenith with the heavy dub which poured out of London and Kingston in the mid to late seventies. Bob Marley, who did much to spread the word about Jamaican music with his commercial pop-tinged reggae, also helped open up many people's minds to the beliefs behind Rastafarianism, particularly in Britain.

Their locks were of utmost importance to the Rastas, and a familiar term of abuse was coined in 1974: 'baldhead'. To quote Dick Hebdige in *Subculture*, 1979, 'It refers literally to those who don't wear "dreadlocks", but can be used to designate all the "sinners" who remain tied to Babylon'. For many whites, this Rasta scene was extremely enticing, not least for punks. 'Dread, in particular, was an enviable commodity,' says Hebdige. 'It was the means with which to menace, and the elaborate freemasonry through which it was sustained and communicated on the street – the colours, the locks, the patois – was awesome and forbidding, suggesting as it did an impregnable solidarity, an asceticism born of suffering.'

As Rasta and reggae became fashionable, so they both began to be amalgamated into the polysynthetic world of the late seventies and early eighties subculture in Britain. There was a ska revival, an indigenous reggae revival, bands like Madness, The Police and Scritti Politti mixed reggae with pop, people began wearing short locks, manicured locks, white locks, false locks, Japanese dreads, funki dreads.

Superdread Bob Marley.

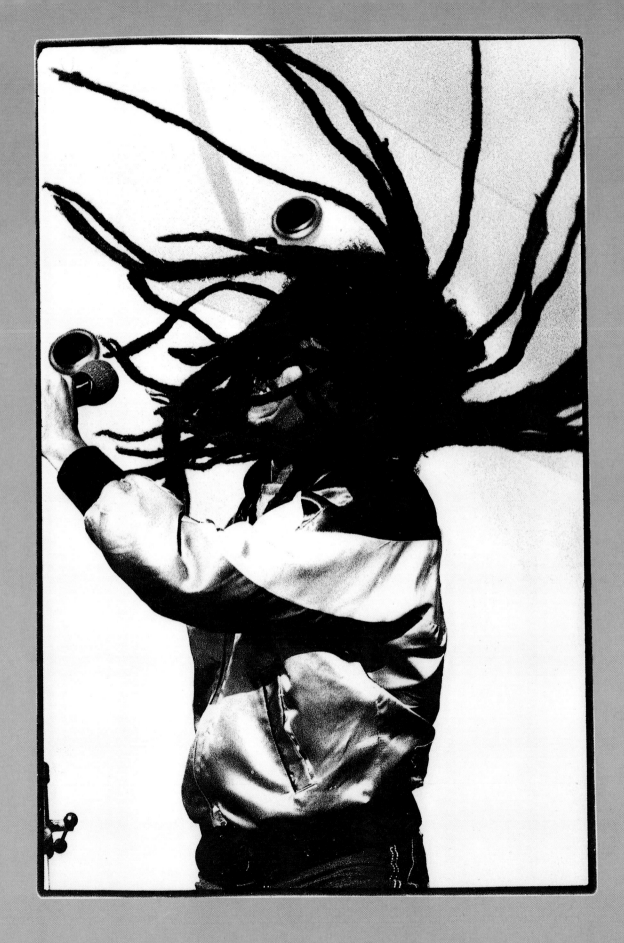

tree!

David Hinds' Tower of Strength

As the leader of seminal British reggae band Steel Pulse, David Hinds has always been a compelling performer and outspoken lyricist. A devout follower of Rastafari, in 1981 Hinds decided to mould his locks into a tall tree of hair, apeing some of the more flamboyant styles of the early Jamaican Rastas. Part of Hinds's stage outfit during Steel Pulse's 1980 and 1981 tours was a bowler hat, and after several months of wearing it, his hair began to take its shape. 'It was then,' he says, 'that I decided to try and grow it all the way up. My hair is an expression of my devotion to the Rastafari faith, and I get a lot of respect from other Rastas because of it. My hair is religious, cultural, not fashionable.'

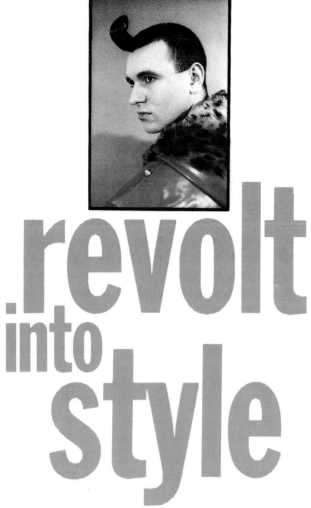

revolt
into
style

In the style-obsessed eighties the world became a global catwalk. Narcissism plumbed new depths as haircuts reached new heights. The eighties rapidly became the designer decade, where everyone had an alias, an ambition and an aerodynamic haircut to match.

Rockabillies spawned psychobillies as the New Romantics gave birth to D.I.Y. mutants and the nightclubs of the western world filled with a new generation of fashion victim. In the controlled chaos of the decade, the haircult reigned.

the new romantics

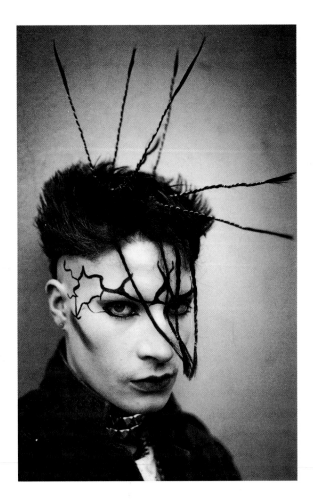

Back to the Future

'New romantics' was the journalistic tag given to the group of bright young things who began to appear in trendy London nightclubs at the end of the seventies. The fashion and music worlds suddenly went mad as everybody under the age of thirty (and some a bit over) realized that if they wanted their fifteen minutes of fame, they'd better take them soon. Image became more important than content, and pop stars began furiously reinventing themselves, as everyone did the resurrection shuffle. They came, they saw, they photocopied.

The Blitz generation took punk and dressed it up, gave it a twelve-inch dance remix and styled its hair. This was skip culture, where something old, something new and something borrowed were all used to create the emperor's new clothes. The new romantics scrambled the codes so much that at first people had difficulty putting a label on this new youth cult, and suggested things like the 'now crowd', 'peacock punks' and 'blitz kids' before settling on new romantics. They were the cult with no name, but with plenty of trousers.

The age of plunder had arrived, and as period dress became fashionable, Britain experienced a haircut revolution as past, present and future were all pushed into one giant gender blender. What came out the other end was entirely up to you: a geometric thatch, a constructivist quiff, a spiralling wedge, a peroxide beehive, a George Orwell cut – the haircut could be palm tree or car crash. With a quick snip of the scissors and the right Rebel Gel you could be who you wanted to be: Clark Kent or Mary Queen of Scots, Captain Kirk or James Dean.

Spandau Ballet were the original new romantic band, the urban village's own pop group, and their robotic, kinetic dance-pop quickly became the soundtrack of 1980. Their mutant wedges and quiffs were soon seen as the quintessential haircuts of the time, and were constantly copied.

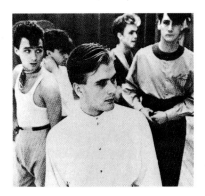

Opposite:Anabella Lwin of Bow Wow Wow. Anglo-Burmese punk with glamorous feline Apache. In Bow Wow Wow, manager Malcolm McLaren tried to combine Burundi punk rock with adolescent fantasies of forbidden sex (Anabella was only 14 years old when she was recruited for the group); seeing as they only had two Top Ten hits in their four year career, the former Sex Pistols svengali was only partially successful.

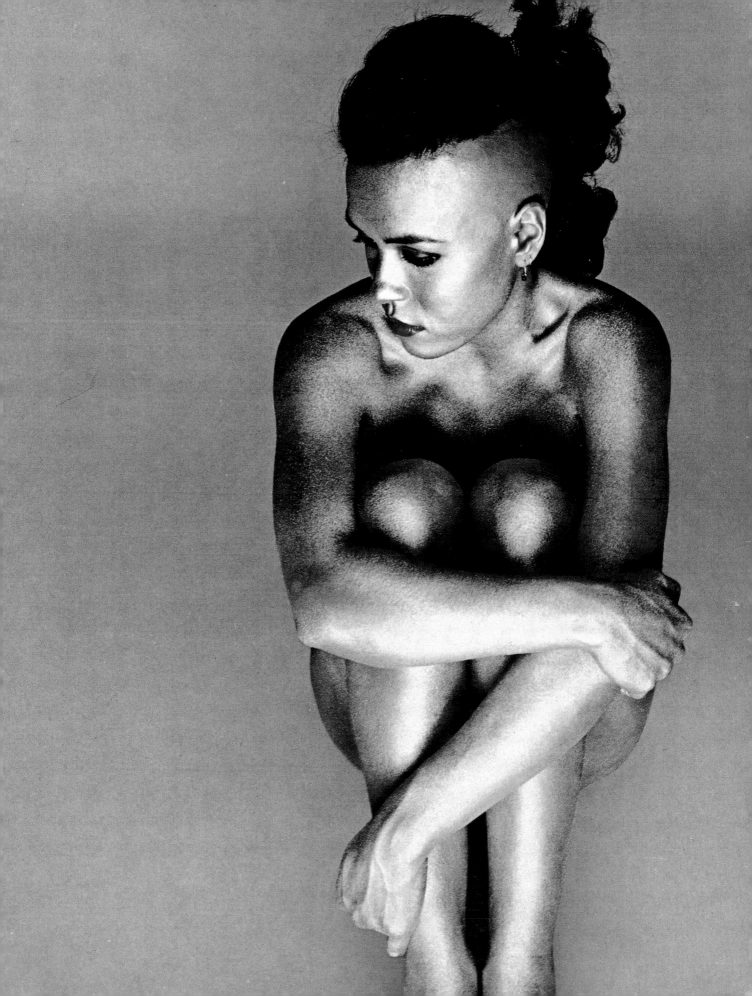

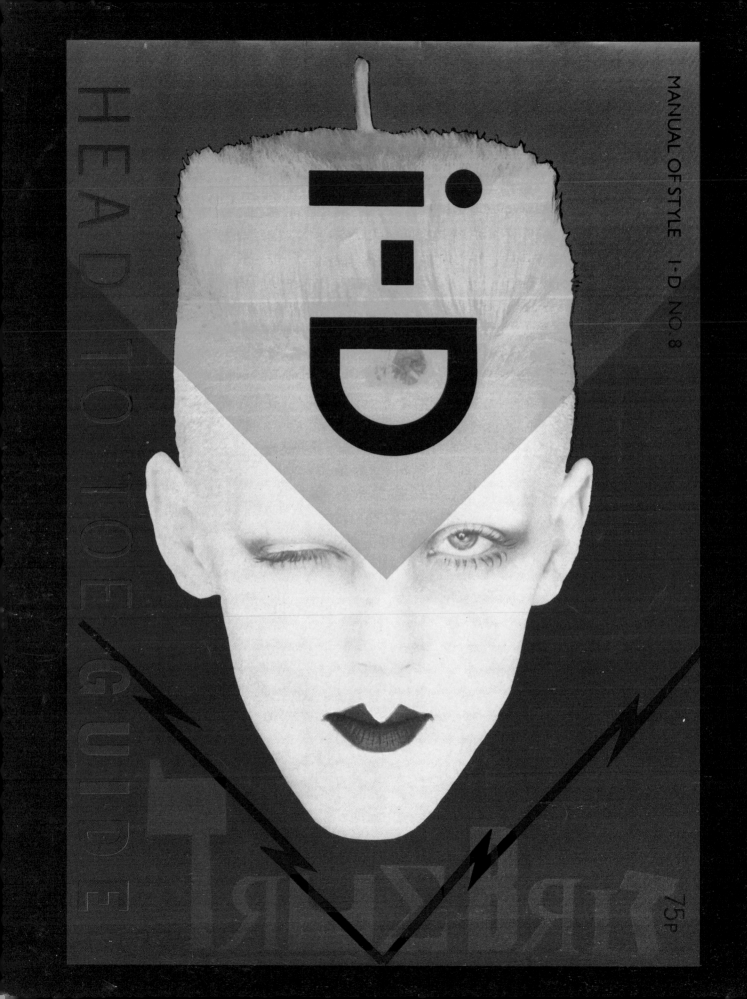

MANUAL OF STYLE I·D NO. 8

HEAD TO TOE GUIDE

75P

the blitz kids

1980 was the year in which the Blitz Kids embroiled themselves in all kinds of religious imagery, donning nuns's habits, outsized crucifixes and deathly white make-up. As far as they were concerned, religion was just another taboo waiting to be broken. The Blitz Kids made their first appearance en masse at the St. Martin's School of Art's second Alternative Fashion Show in May 1980, partly inspired by Boy George, and were ceremoniously applauded and then pelted by the crowd. Here, Antenna hairdresser and sometime model Scarlett sports a hair crucifix.

Left: The front cover of *i-D* No.8, Spring, 1982; Scarlett again, this time with a tall peroxide flat top, with additional apple stalk. Like the sixties, when long hair would be entwined with graphics on LP sleeves – *Disraeli Gears* and *Revolver* spring to mind – to fake a sense of spiritual or mystical rebellion, so this image is similarly enhanced by a striking use of graphics and colour, albeit implying rather different sentiments.

I-D PHOTOGRAPHER THOMAS DEGEN SNAPPED 'PEACE PAINTING' IN MUNICH AND CRUCIFIX CUTS IN LONDON. PRIMITIVE BUT POWERFUL, THE CURRENT 'OVER THE TOP' FACE PAINTING WITNESSES EARTHY HIPPYS AND DEDICATED FOLLOWERS OF PSYCHEDELIA CONFUSING FASHION AND SUPPOSED ANTI-FASHION AS NEVER BEFORE.

RUCIFIX CUT WORN BY SCARLETT – ANTENNAE.

Make-up!

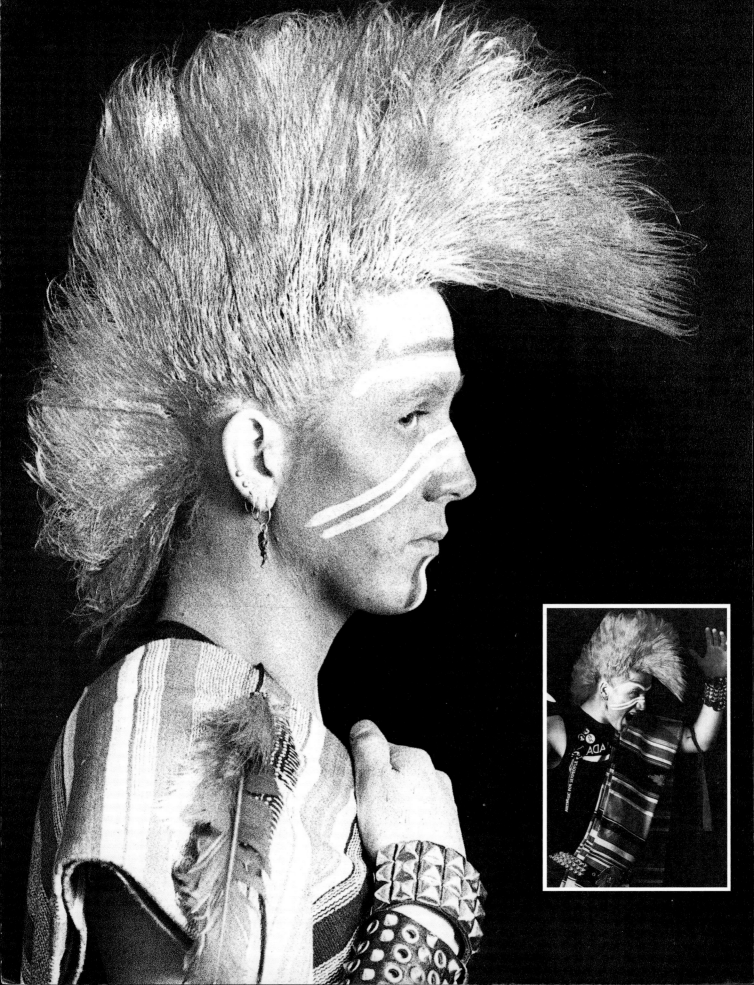

kingfisher

steve strange

Incensed at a photo story concerning nightclub socialite Steve Strange, his wacky friends, lifestyle, clothes, make-up and haircut, which appeared in *The Face* in October 1980, an irate reader calling himself Mitch wrote to the magazine explaining his own idiosyncratic haircut. 'Please find enclosed,' he wrote, 'two shots of what I claim to be the most famous original hairstyle in Britain, maybe even the world. The Kingfisher cut, created two months ago by me, is basically two massive fins growing on each side of my head and meeting at the front, with the middle being hollow. The first shot shows my reaction to Steve Strange after seeing his pathetic attempt at ripping me off. The second picture is the Kingfisher finally realizing that his hairstyle is so brilliant that no one could ever successfully copy it. Mitch (The Kingfisher), South Moor, Stanley, Co. Durham.'

This was a typical attitude of the eighties. Everyone wanted a different look to everyone else – one week it was space age, the next it was the Louis Quatorze look, zoot-suited gangsters the next. Punks, new romantics, gothics, rockabillies, none of them wanted exactly the same haircut, and one-up-manship became the predictable raison d'être for most nightclub denizens. There was little bonhomie, and it was every haircut for himself.

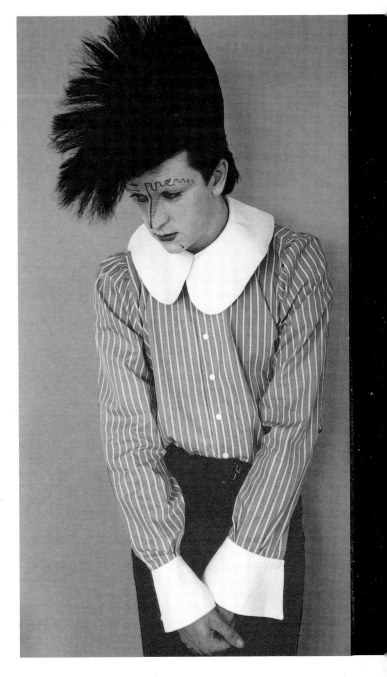

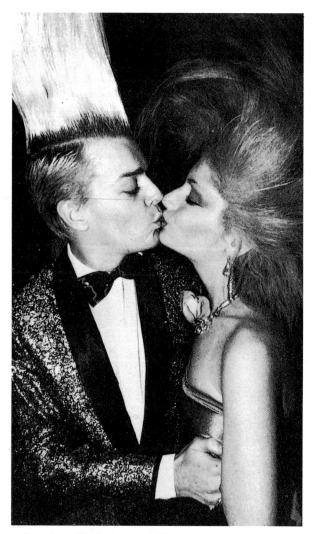

Downtown Manhattan socialite John Sex, pictured in 1984.

humanoid

Human League singer Phil Oakey had the perfect post-modernist haircut for the perfect post-modernist pop group of 1981. Always Sheffield's finest exponents of ironic-pop (as art school pranksters in the late seventies the League had toyed with rickety indie-pop and split-screen slide shows), this regrouped band of post-pop/post-modern futurists (the meaningless tags of eighties dancehall pop) embraced three minute synth-pop and fashion house imagery. Throughout these changes one thing remained constant – Oakey's ridiculous 'piste', a haircut short on one side and long on the other. He has been quoted as saying that the only reason he had it cut this way was the hope it would get him, and the band, noticed.

hair today, gone today

By the mid eighties fledgling pop stars were using all kinds of weird haircuts as a means of getting themselves noticed by the press. No longer was a particular haircut representative of a particular group of people and if, in a nightclub, you bumped into someone with a gigantic sixteen-inch charcoal-black conk, it by no means meant that they had anything to do with rock'n'roll; PR was probably their game.

As their meanings became more confused, more diffused, as their codes became scrambled, so haircuts became more idiosyncratic, losing some symbolic importance on the way. The legacy is still with us, and a visit to Portobello Road or Kensington Market in London, the Lower East Side in New York, Venice Beach in Los Angeles, in fact anywhere in the western world with access to a radio and a pair of scissors and you will come across the muted death-knell of punk rock, living on in dirty black denim, gothic costume jewellery and matted, partially shaved peroxide dreadlocks, or a combination of some or all of these. These days, rebellion is on a life-support system.

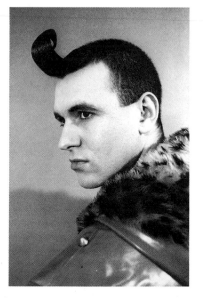

Babytime! ABC's Mark White's heavily lacquered postmodern cartoon of the Tin-Tin quiff was a blatant copy of the munchkin haircut in Victor Fleming's 1939 version of *The Wizard of Oz*.

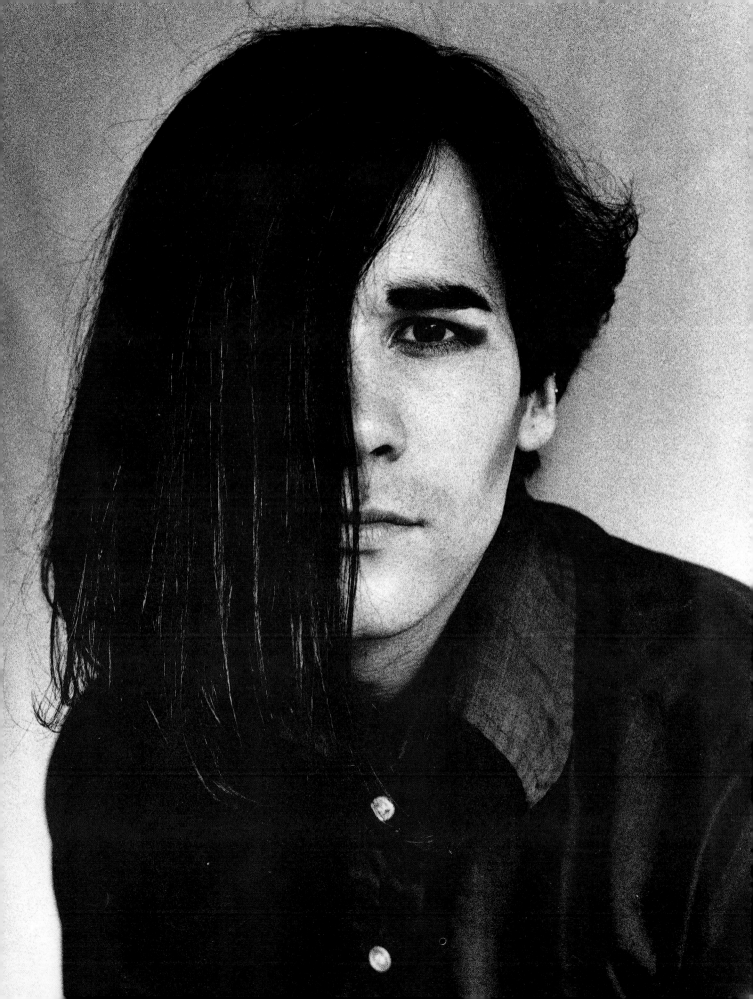

antenna

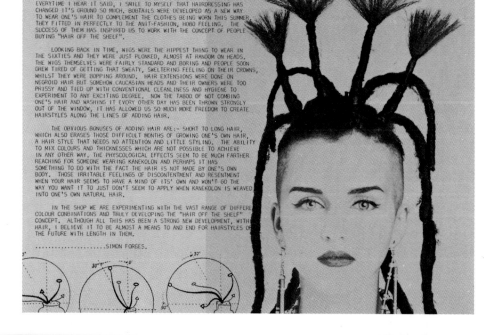

"THINK I'LL GET MY HAIR LENGTHENED"

THIS IS A PHRASE I HEAR FREQUENTLY IN ANTENNA THESE DAYS AND EVERYTIME I HEAR IT SAID, I SMILE TO MYSELF THAT HAIRDRESSING HAS CHANGED IT'S GROUND SO MUCH. BOBTAILS WERE DEVELOPED AS A NEW WAY TO WEAR ONE'S HAIR TO COMPLEMENT THE CLOTHES BEING WORN THIS SUMMER. THEY FITTED IN PERFECTLY TO THE ANTI-FASHION, HOBO FEELING. THE SUCCESS OF THEM HAS INSPIRED US TO WORK WITH THE CONCEPT OF PEOPLE BUYING "HAIR OFF THE SHELF".

LOOKING BACK IN TIME, WIGS WERE THE HIPPEST THING TO WEAR IN THE SIXTIES AND THEY WERE JUST PLONKED, ALMOST AT RANDOM ON HEADS. THE WIGS THEMSELVES WERE FAIRLY STANDARD AND BORING AND PEOPLE SOON GREW TIRED OF GETTING THAT SWEATY, SWELTERING FEELING ON THEIR CROWNS, WHILST THEY WERE BOPPING AROUND. HAIR EXTENSIONS WERE DONE ON NEGROID HAIR BUT SOMEHOW CAUCASIAN HEADS AND THEIR OWNERS WERE TOO PRISSY AND TIED UP WITH CONVENTIONAL CLEANLINESS AND HYGIENE TO EXPERIMENT TO ANY EXCITING DEGREE. NOW THE TABOO OF NOT COMBING ONE'S HAIR AND WASHING IT EVERY OTHER DAY HAS BEEN THROWN STRONGLY OUT OF THE WINDOW, IT HAS ALLOWED US SO MUCH MORE FREEDOM TO CREATE HAIRSTYLES ALONG THE LINES OF ADDING HAIR.

THE OBVIOUS BONUSES OF ADDING HAIR ARE:- SHORT TO LONG HAIR, WHICH ALSO ERASES THOSE DIFFICULT MONTHS OF GROWING ONE'S OWN HAIR, A HAIR STYLE THAT NEEDS NO ATTENTION AND LITTLE STYLING. THE ABILITY TO MIX COLOURS AND THICKNESSES WHICH ARE NOT POSSIBLE TO ACHIEVE IN ANY OTHER WAY, THE PHYSCOLOGICAL EFFECTS SEEM TO BE MUCH FARTHER REACHING FOR SOMEONE WEARING KANEKOLON AND PERHAPS IT HAS SOMETHING TO DO WITH THE FACT THE HAIR IS NOT MADE BY ONE'S OWN BODY. THOSE IRRITABLE FEELINGS OF DISCONTENTMENT AND RESENTMENT WHEN YOUR HAIR SEEMS TO HAVE A MIND OF ITS' OWN AND WON'T GO THE WAY YOU WANT IT TO JUST DON'T SEEM TO APPLY WHEN KANEKOLON IS WEAVED INTO ONE'S OWN NATURAL HAIR.

IN THE SHOP WE ARE EXPERIMENTING WITH THE VAST RANGE OF DIFFERENT COLOUR COMBINATIONS AND TRULY DEVELOPING THE "HAIR OFF THE SHELF" CONCEPT. ALTHOUGH ALL THIS HAS BEEN A STRONG NEW DEVELOPMENT, WITH HAIR, I BELIEVE IT TO BE ALMOST A MEANS TO AND END FOR HAIRSTYLES OF THE FUTURE WITH LENGTH IN THEM.

.................SIMON FORBES.

A creative director for Alan International from 1971 to 1979, in July 1980 Simon Forbes opened his own hair salon, Antenna. A reflection of London's haircut revolution, Forbes soon began developing hair extensions, as well as a range of colouring techniques, and in 1981 introduced monofibre. Artificial hair of the highest calibre, monofibre helped Forbes create many styles of hair extensions, including bobtails, ragtails, warlocks, cable curls, frizettes and spindlelocks.

bobtails

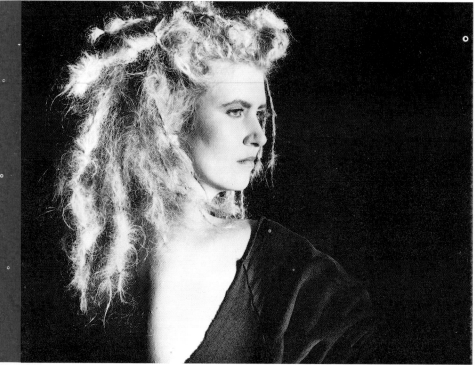

Dateline February 1982: Antenna's bobtails, or white dreadlocks, were introduced, according to Forbes, 'to cater for the demand for casual, sexy and untidy hairstyles . . . for the anti-fashion, hobo feeling.' This was really Hair Off The Shelf, the first time any hairdresser had attempted such a thing. 'Now the taboo of not combing one's hair and washing it every other day has been thrown strongly out of the window.' Here the hair has been shaved into a mohawk, with bobtails added in two different shades, cut and fanned to give an antennae effect.

ragtails

Dateline September 1982: after bobtails, Simon Forbes introduced ragtails – pieces of real and false hair, combed or matted but not necessarily 'locked', woven into the customer's own thatch.

boy george

Culture Club were originally a mish-mash of sexual, cultural, stylistic and musical codes. The dreadlocks of George O'Dowd were neither deferential nor iconoclastic – but they were shocking and, in hindsight, completely appropriate for the times. George was never a white Rasta, more a sartorial jigsaw puzzle. In January 1982 he told *New Sounds New Styles*, 'I'm not at all religious; I think the dreadlocks look good and the star (of David) is a nice symbol. People take symbolism too seriously(!). Basically, I wear it to annoy people.' Boy George on the cover of Culture Club's first single, 'White Boy', Virgin, 1982).

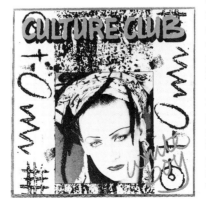

head start

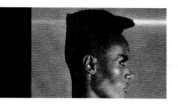

In 1985, on behalf of Citroën, French advertising agency RSCG commissioned Jean-Paul Goude to design a poster campaign for their new CX GTI Turbo. Using the increasingly accommodating Grace Jones he created 'the world's first wind-tunnel-tested D.A.'. Jones was also used by Goude in the TV advertising which followed this campaign.

amazing grace

Grace Jones was a highly successful model struggling as a highly unsuccessful singer until she met French art director Jean-Paul Goude. In the early seventies Grace, along with fellow American Jerry Hall, enchanted the catwalks of Paris with her fine features (the Jones Bones) and sleek ebony body, rapidly becoming the fashion industry's most sought after black model. In 1977 she began singing, subsequently signing for Island Records, where she recorded a series of lame gay disco LPs before taking up with Goude.

Together they worked on hundreds of portraits of Grace, exploiting her sexuality in a variety of colourful and subversive images, usually involving montage or photorealistic techniques. The result of this was the reinvention of Grace Jones as 'the first black new wave artist', the combination of enticing androgyny and rarified Fourth World Funk perfectly capturing the spirit of 1980.

processed hair

It is said that the straightening of hair for black people was initiated about a hundred years ago by Madam C.J. Walker, a Pittsburgh woman who invented the original straightening comb (a heated fork had been used up until then) and who also opened one of the first American beauty colleges. Women began straightening their naturally curly hair to make it more manageable, but the look soon became a desirable style. Not to be outdone, the men developed the conk in the twenties. Chemicals were later invented which could be used to straighten the hair, but even though the method was usually laborious, as the black population of America grew, so did the 'process'.

Hair straightening became part of everyday life for most black Americans, and even continued in popularity throughout the sixties and seventies, when black America made its cultural, psychological and philosophical migration to Africa. In the eighties there has been a revolution in black hairdressing, particularly in America, and there are now hundreds of different ways of wearing black hair.

The first person to open a hair straightening salon in Britain (to cater for the first-generation immigrants) was a 38-year-old Trinidadian Carmen Maingot. Her Kensington hairdressers opened in May 1955.

Some people still feel that processed hair of any kind signifies black assimilation into white society. Film director Spike Lee finds this ridiculous: in *School Daze* (1988) he explores the theme of black racial division by focusing on the rifts and rivalries between a group of wannabees and jigaboos in an all-black American college. Needless to say, the wannabees have processed hair and the jigaboos don't. At the time of the film's release he said, 'I think it's going to bother a whole lot of black people. Not that they don't know it's true. It's the fact that it's being exposed for the world to see that will bother them. But I hope they will come to the realization that there are too many things which keep us divided.'

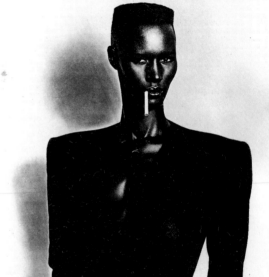

This classic silhouette can be best seen on the cover of her 1981 LP *Nightclubbing*.

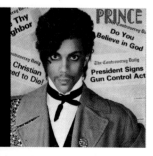

Prince on the cover of his *Controversy* LP (1981), wearing highly-styled processed hair.

On the cover of her *Living My Life* LP (1982) Grace's hair was exaggerated even more. Now it was geometrically perfect, a counterfeit illusion with not a hair out of place. Her femininity was altered still more, the vorticist profile, bloodshot eyes, airbrushed sweatbeads and tactically placed boxer's plaster all furthering her androgynous image as the woman in the iron mask.

Grace Jones had some strange attributes – her gigantic men's Armani jackets, her robotic way of dancing, and her raspy, slow drawl. But the most startling thing about her was her magnificent pill-box flat-top (which had begun life on Goude's drawing board), a haircut of high geometric absurdity. It quickly spread: for Jones's 'One Man Show', a live revue which toured Europe in 1982, Goude enlisted the help of a dozen Jones Clones, a gaggle of equally lithe models all sporting the laser-sculpted bell-hop cut. This masterful creation was a fashion victim's delight, and soon nightclubs all over the world were full of animatronic Jones clones, all with immaculately chiselled flat-tops and menacing, if overly camp stares.

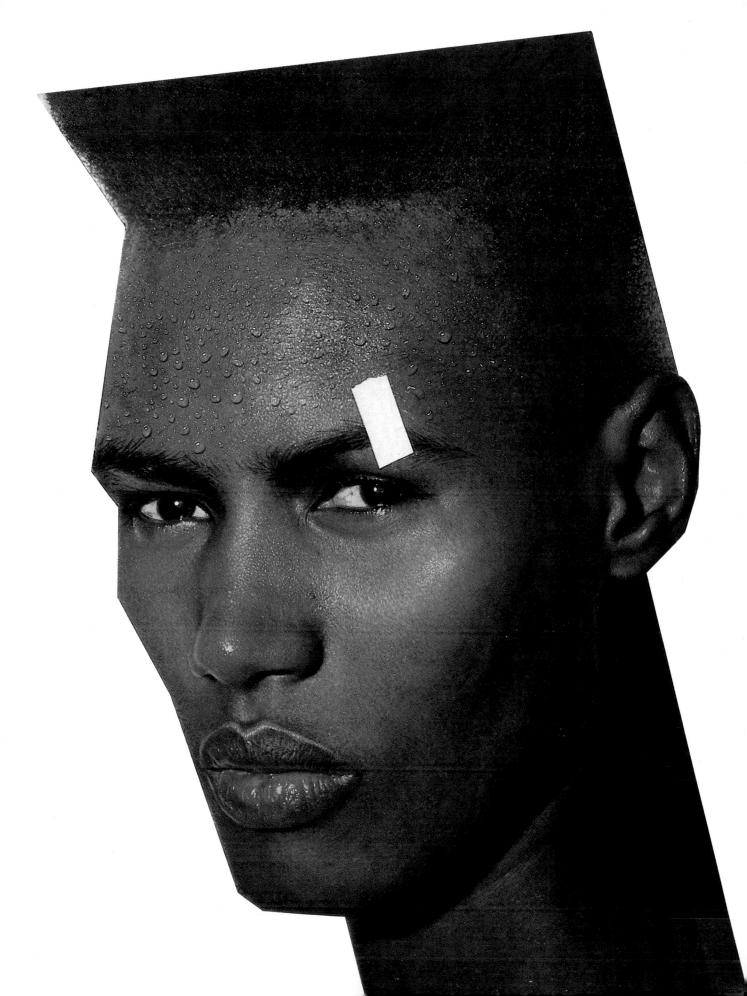

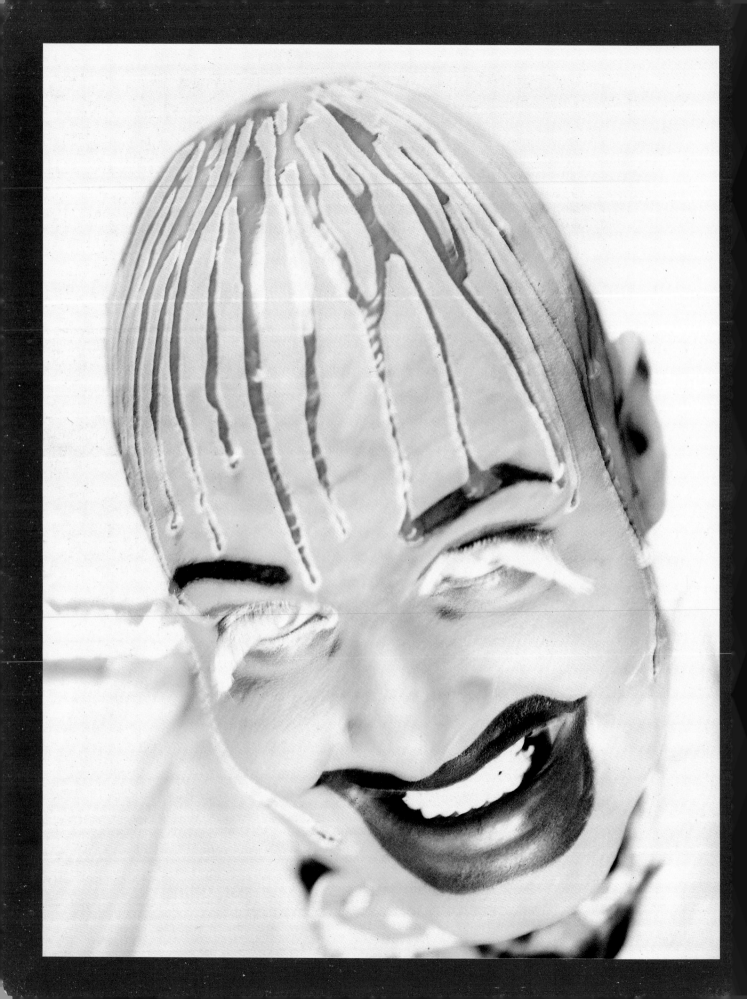

leigh bowery

After Dame Edna Everage, Leigh Bowery is Australia's most celebtrated eccentric and least likely cultural attaché. An emigrant from a small suburb of Melbourne called Sunshine, Leigh made his name in London in the mid eighties through his outrageous way of dressing. He has been fashion designer, club runner and dancer, but it is for his dress sense that he became famous.

As a regular fixture of London clubland he was seen in so many weird and wonderful creations that he became a fashion icon in himself. Leigh would one night be the Statue of Liberty, a herpes virus, glam stormtrooper or imploded meringue. Leigh made fashion victims quake in their mauve, velveteen platform boots, because not only did he outshine all of them, he also constantly reinvented himself, with little regard for ego or perceptions of taste.

Leigh became a constantly changing hologram; to quote Alix Sharkey, 'He was no longer a designer but a design. He transcended fashion and became something else, closer to the imagery of 'pop surrealist' painters like Kenny Scharf. Leigh Bowery had become a cartoon character, less than human but larger than life.'

Leigh once appeared on the cover of a magazine as a pig – wearing three pairs of spectacles, foam ears, and a tiny pigtail atop his crown.

Perhaps Leigh's greatest invention was his cracked egg, a bald dome with different kinds of wax poured over it. For Leigh this look was extremely popular, and he spent most of 1986 looking as though someone had just spilt a bottle of ink over his cranium.

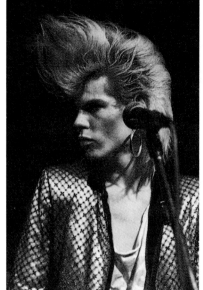

Sigue Sigue Sputnik's resident mega-quiff, Neal X.

sigue sigue sputnik

The brainchild of ex-Generation X guitarist Tony James, Sigue Sigue Sputnik (their name taken from a Moscow street gang) were a glorious, vacuous scam, the world's first complete science-fiction pop group. Employing the services of fully-fledged fashion victim Martin Degville, fashion designer and haircut about town, James set about creating a brash reaction against the antiseptic quality of eighties pop, in a severely tainted re-run of punk. According to James, music had become just another accessory in the lifestyle explosion we were all supposed to embrace.

Sputnik were meant to shock us out of our complacency, with visions of designer violence, gaudy hi-tech glamour (reminiscent of the New York Dolls), cod-Japanese techno-babble and manic computerized rock 'n' roll. The group was to be the flagship of a corporate youth cult for the post-industrial age, but though they had some initial success with their single 'Love Missile F1-11', ultimately Sigue Sigue Sputnik were found to be firing blanks. 'It was Martin Degville who really encapsulated the way the band should look', says James. 'When I first met him – in the basement of Kensington Market in 1982 – he looked like nothing on earth, he had waist-length blonde dreadlocks (Degville made his locks out of carpets and hearthrugs), with one side of his head shaved, dancing to Suicide records in white stilettos and a red PVC mini skirt. The eventual package was far better than my original idea' – Degville helped with both James' pink pineapple and Neal's global quiff – 'though we had to wait for the talent to catch up with the haircuts. I think if people look brilliant then they'll eventually be able to play . . . but it's more difficult to make a good musician look good. You can teach people to be good singers but you can't teach them to be thin. In a way we created our own deathtrap because the image was so strong. Things are so much more accelerated these days – Bowie was allowed to use Ziggy's haircut for three albums (actually four), but we were only allowed one.'

'Sigue Sigue Sputnik – They're weird, they're wonderful, and they're swindling their way to the top!' (*The Sun*)

a close shave

logomania!

1987 was the year when the bastions of London street fashion became intoxicated by conspicous consumption, brazenly wearing fake designer logos on T-shirts, MA1 flying jackets, baseball caps and b-boy name belts, etc; relatively cheap items of clothing which not only commandeered the labels of upmarket shopping (Chanel, Gucci, Hermes, Louis Vuitton), but in the process rendered them meaningless, and stripped of status.

This bootlegging fascination also stretched to the logos of certain makes of car, the most popular being Volkswagen, BMW and Mercedes. During the summer months, so many hubcaps and metal logos were stolen from parked Volkswagens (and subsequently worn around the neck on metal chains by the new owners – mostly teenage Beastie Boys fans) that the manufacturers offered to supply any prospective owner (i.e. the bootleggers themselves) with a replica of the VW logo. The tiny steel badge (25mm in diameter, as opposed to the 76mm version, which was only supplied to genuine VW owners) came with a rather patronising covering letter hoping that 'one day you might be able to buy the car to go with the badge!' Needless to say this didn't stop the mass theft of hubcaps, though by the winter the craze had petered out.

Opposite page: **Some hip-hop afficionados took their allegiance just that little bit further, having the VW logo shaved into their heads, while others exhibited a fondness for designer themes.**

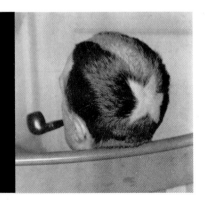

Partially shaving the head has always had immense shock value, particularly when combined with what appears to be highly conventional costume. 'Tonsure', from 1921, is a photograph of Marcel Duchamp by Man Ray showing a star cut into the back of the Dadaist's head, recalling the hairstyle of Catholic priests in a symbol of self-castration.

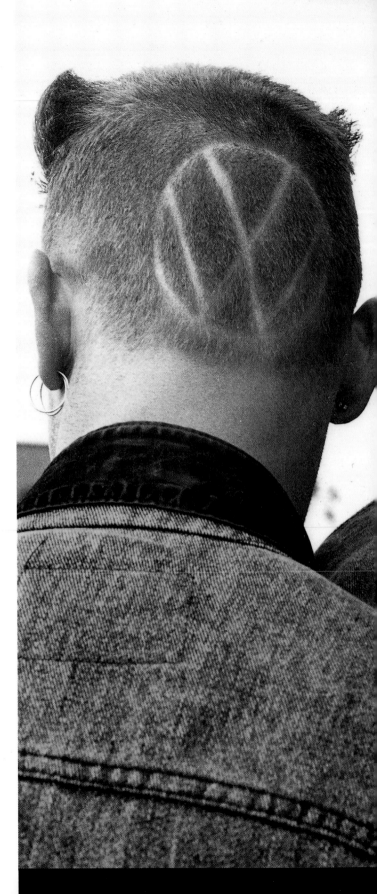

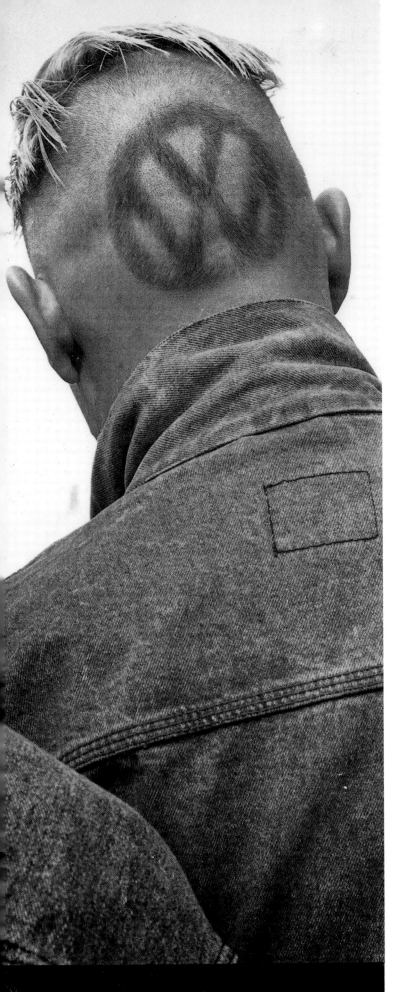

In the frantic run-up to Superbowl '88, the States' most celebrated sporting event, team tribalism was taken to extremes in New Orleans. The local football team, perennial NFC losers the Saints, were suddenly winning every game they played and the whole city was seething with what became known as Saintsmania. The team's emblem, a black Fleur de Lys (New Orleans is a French town), was omnipresent, with diehards like the supporter shown here proudly shaving their tribal markings into their hair. Note the shaved rings, making the emblem even more prominent.

saints mania

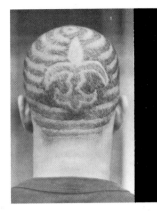

b-boy style

The emergence of hip-hop culture in New York in the late seventies, the mass adoption of rap music, scratch DJs, breakdancing styles and graffiti art by the South Bronx's indigenous black youth, prompted a definite style of dress for the emergent b-boys and fly-girls. Labelled sportswear – Adidas, Kangol, Nike, Fila, Le Coq Sportif, Puma, etc. – became *de rigeur*, as did closely cropped hair and baseball caps. About the only fashion accessory from the excessive seventies which stayed the course was gold, resplendent in oversized jewellery. The first real superstars of hip-hop — the first rap merchants to make it to the stadiums — were Run DMC, who took sponsorship to new heights by recording a single called 'My Adidas'.

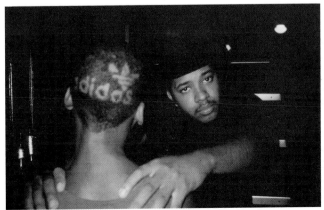

Here a young b-boy shows his allegiance to the band, having the Adidas logo shaved into his scalp.

braids

Braids and cornrows have been popular as hairstyles with African women for as long as anyone can remember; African sculptures from as far back as 900 B.C. show women wearing both styles. When Africans were brought to America as slaves, women continued to wear their hair this way. During the years which followed, as American blacks began straightening their hair in approximations of white styles, braiding and cornrows began to take on increasing cultural significance.

During black America's nationalist resurgence in the late sixties and early seventies, braids replaced the Afro as the ultimate haircut of emancipation. *Time* devoted a piece to the waning popularity of the Afro in its 25 October issue in 1971, quoting a hipper than thou black politician as saying, 'Afros are as out of date as plantation bandanas'. *Time* may have had an interest in defusing such a radical symbol as the Afro, but it is certain that by this time more young blacks were wearing neo-African braids, plaits and variations of cornrows.

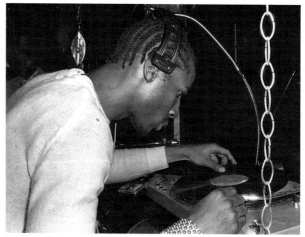

DJ Grandmaster Flash on his wheels of steel at New York's Broadway International in 1984, sporting skull-hugging cornrows.

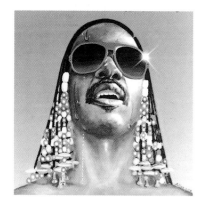

Stevie Wonder as he appears on the cover of his 1980 Motown LP *Hotter Than July*.

In Africa, braids have been as much of a utilitarian style as anything else (the shorter cornrows were mostly worn by children), and though the connotations today are different, utility is still important. After the initial braiding process the hair can be left for over two months before it needs attention (something which can't be said for chemically processed hair). Forty years ago, braids were also an interim stage in the hair styling process. According to Ruth Houston, a contributing editor at *Black Elegance*, 'The black woman who was going to press and curl her hair, shampooed it, then braided it up until she was ready for that process.'

Braiding is relatively simple – basically the intertwining of three pieces of hair – but today as its popularity grows, and salons spring up across the United States, new styles involving braiding and cornrows have evolved, from the basket-weave and the French roll to the twist, the crimp or simple braided bob. Braiding is also enjoying massive popularity because of the increased awareness that hair can be irreparably damaged by the application of too many chemicals. (Many specialist hairdressers also claim that braiding is therapeutic.)

bam

Afrika Bambaataa is the self-proclaimed leader of the Zulu Nation, a loosely constructed organization dedicated to education, peace and survival among Bambaataa's fellow south-east Bronx comrades. Bambaataa (the name of a nineteenth-century Zulu chief, meaning Chief Affection), or Bam as he is more commonly known, was a figurehead for many wayward black youths in New York during the late seventies and early eighties. His most famous hairstyle was his black Mohican, later adopted by the *A-Team*'s Mr T. 'It was punk which made me do it,' says Bambaataa, 'I saw all those white kids with their Mohawks and it made me jealous. So I went to see my friend Claude, who's got a little barbershop down in the South Bronx, and he cut me a real fine one, the first black one of its kind. People say it looks violent, but they've got the wrong idea. It's meant to look tribal, strong, a feature of the Zulu Nation. It just looks funky to me . . .' Bambaataa was also renowned for the thin razored lines across the sides of his head, a style which would later be copied by countless b-boys.

the philly cut

The Philly cut is an appropriation of a thirties style called a tapered cut, which was popular with Philadelphia Muslims. There were two lengths – a high 'English' and a low 'English', meaning a high taper or a low taper, though both looked like a black crew cut, a style which also became popular with many blacks who didn't belong to the Muslim religion. Philadelphia was a popular place of visit for blacks from Washington D.C. (not least because of work), and one of the things they brought back to 'Chocolate City' was the Philly cut.

During the seventies the haircut became more extreme, distinguishing itself from the Black Muslim natural. The new Philly cut was more accentuated, like a black signet ring, with sharp edges and high tops. In the eighties the hairstyle has been associated with the many Go-Go groups which have sprung up in Washington. A mobile, percussive funk music, propelled by a double-edged rhythm, Go-Go went global in 1983–84, and bands like Trouble Funk, Chuck Brown & The Soul Searchers and Redds & The Boys, started to receive worldwide exposure, taking the Philly cut with them.

Recently the Philly has become a catch-all phrase which covers everything from a skinhead cut which has grown out on top, to a sculpted Afro, like those worn by Grace Jones or Larry Blackmon from funk group Cameo. These days it's not unusual to see young black kids with many parallel cuts shaved into their heads just above the ears, or with long tapered Vs at the back. Olympic sprinter Carl Lewis and boxer Mike Tyson have both worn Philly cuts at some stage in their careers.

Trouble Funk: the Philly cut goes Go-Go.

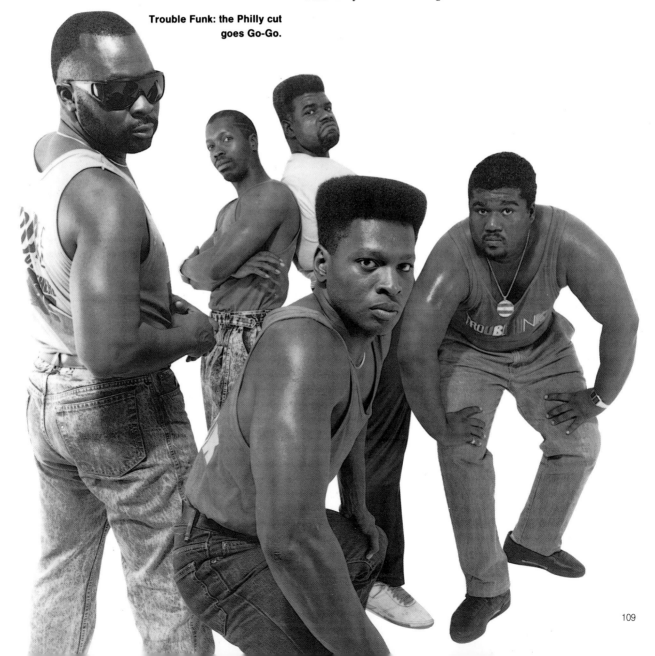

revolt into style

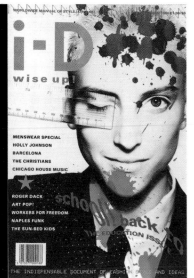

Amanda King.

During 1976–77, nothing was more confrontational than a bright peroxide crop, a blonde spiky-top glistening with hairspray. Five years later and this style had been completely devoured by the British high street. First it became a staple for young fashionable girls, and was quickly adopted by post-casual and pre-designer 'terrace tearaways', as well as the young whizz kids of the City. Nowadays it isn't unusual to see young dealers in London's Square Mile sporting bright yellow tufts of heavily gelled hair above their Thomas Pink shirts, woven silk ties and Austin Reed suits.

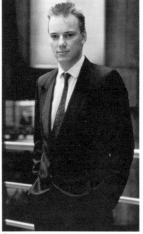

City Boy.

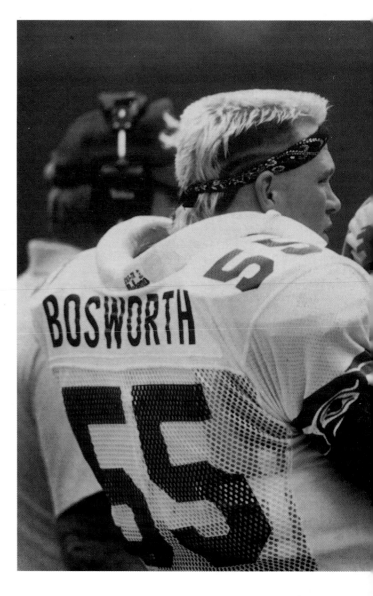

In the summer of 1987 the biggest craze in Milan was the Ruud Gullit baseball cap, a homage to the city's favourite rastafarian. The Dutch striker was the 1986/87 European Footballer of the Year, for whom AC Milan paid PSV Eindhoven nearly £6m. The synthetic dreadlocks unfortunately made anyone who wore the cap look like Ralph, the canine pianist in *The Muppets*, but then it was certainly better than wearing a cap adorned with a Claus Oldenberg hammer, puppy poop, or two cans of Budweiser. This was the ultimate Ruud boy cap.

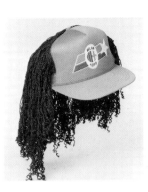

sporting locks

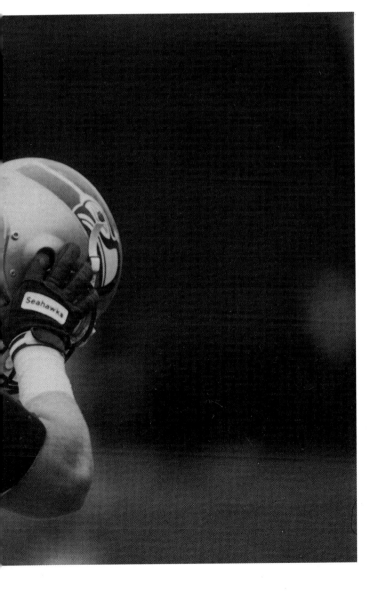

In 1990 the expressive, excessive haircut is no longer the tool of the unruly and the iconoclastic. Today, a 'funny' haircut can be worn by anyone, its impact diminished through years of numbing exposure. Also, although today's haircuts are no less spectacular than they were, say, ten years ago, they express efficiency and energy – haircuts these days are more than likely to have functional qualities as well as being stylistic codes.

This is most evident in the world of sports. Boxers, swimmers, footballers and athletes of all types have taken to their hair with a vengeance. By cutting, shaving and dyeing their hair they are highlighting their idiosyncratic skills, while at the same time making themselves more appealing in the eyes of the world's increasingly rapacious media. Sportsmen use their haircuts to get noticed, to become stars.

One such star is the American football player Brian Bosworth, or 'Boz' as he is more commonly known. In 1988, this former University of Oklahoma linebacker became one of the world's richest sportsmen when he signed with Seattle Seahawks for a record $11 million. Just twenty-three, he also became the most famous – read visible – NFL players in America, appearing on The David Letterman Show, doing cameos on MTV, and even writing an outspoken autobiography, *The Boz: Confessions of a Modern Anti-Hero* (1988). But Bosworth is not an anti-hero in the traditional sense; the modern-day version is an aggressive, loudmouthed football player with a larger-than-life, tailored Mohican hairdo. In his book he writes at length about his uncompromising locks, including: 'I don't give a rat's ass what people think about my hair…It's a way to express my individuality. I modify it all the time – long, short, long tail, no tail, different designs and stripes. I don't want anyone getting an edge on me.'

On the body beautiful the Bosworth Mohican looks terrific. It's powerful, proud and sophisticated. It's sleek, it's dynamic, and it's sexy. But these days it's only a haircut, an exercise in style. Chris Savage-King, writing in *The New Statesman/Society* in November 1988, stated: 'That hair's considered our crowning glory isn't incidental. It's both part of our bodies, and part of our decoration. Its condition can denote our health in ways both physical and cultural, yet the current trends veer towards a sleekness that's superficial. For all their invention, they point towards denial.'

Savage-King believes the modern-day haircut to be completely utilitarian, whether it be crew cut or Mohican, though this can be said about the general trends of all fashion during the late eighties. Hairstyles are no less important than they were fifty years ago, but today we seem to have run the gamut of styles, and if not the gamut of styles then certainly the gamut of meaning. The haircut will no doubt be re-invented either out of necessity or fashion for as long as people have hair, though whether there will ever be anything as powerful, as proud, or as sexy as Elvis Presley's blue-black quiff remains to be seen.

Acknowledgments

With very special thanks to Neil Spencer.

Thanks also to Afrika Bambaataa, Steve Beard, Phil Bicker, the British Library, Neville Brody, Stuart Cosgrove, Robin Derrick, Tony Elliott, Jeffrey Ferry, Helen Gallagher, David Hinds, Tony James, Terry Jones, Nick Kent, Nick Knight, Lee Leschasin, Chris Logan, Nick Logan, Tony Peake, Jon Savage, Alix Sharkey, Siouxsie Sioux, Ian Swift, David Toop, Keith Wainwright, Charlotte Wheeler, Simon Witter, Ian Wright, to Audrey and Mike, and especially to Kathryn Flett, without whom, etc.

Picture Credits

t = top; m = middle; b = bottom; l = left; r = right

Ace Records 37m, b   Peter Anderson 29   Mike Owen/Antenna, London 101t   Associated Press 37t   Joe Bangay 86   Patricia Bates 108r   Janette Beckman 28t; 68b; 97   John Benton-Harris 71l   Lynne Franks/Boilerhouse 14; 15; 18   Adrian Boot 88   Billy Boy 41b   Joel Brodsky 62   Camera Press, London 10; 11b Leif Skoogfors; 41r   Harold Chapman 42tr   Charlton Publications 24   Joe Cirello 21   Chris Clunn 107t   Anton Corbijn 99   David Corio 89   Joe Cornish 82   Kevin Cummins 32   Decca 52t   Thomas Degen 94; 95   The Design Museum 80br   EG Records 69   EMI 48mr   Jane England 100t   "Wah Ching Boy, Chinatown, San Francisco, 1969" from IN OUR TIME by Tom Wolfe. Copyright © 1961, 1963, 1964, 1965, 1968, 1971, 1972, 1973, 1975, 1976, 1977, 1978, 1979, 1980 by Tom Wolfe. Reprinted by permission of Farrar, Straus and Giroux, Inc. 34   Hans Feurer 53mr   Galerie Gemurzynska, Cologne 7t   Gifford Wallace Inc. 57l   Phil Stern/Globe Photos 13   Lynn Goldsmith 42b   Jean-Paul Goude 102m, t; 103   Hairdressers' Journal 50b, 79r   Peter Paul Hartnett 105   Heavy Metal Records 74l   History Workshop Journal 12   Hulton-Deutsch 7b; 26l; 27r   Keystone 52br   The Kobal Collection 20   Nick Knight 33; 51; 70t, b; 71t, b; 84; 104; 110t   Barry Lategan 53tr   Patrick Lichfield 52bl   London Features International Ltd 46; 59t   Patsy Louer 106/107   Robert Capa – Magnum 79   Man Ray 8; 106l   Norman Mansbridge 39   de la Mata 28b   Mattel UK Ltd 45   Mike McGrath 60   Dennis Morris 81b   Motown 108l   National Film Archive, London 16; 22; 72t; 76; 78l   New York Daily News 25t   Michael Ochs Archives 26r; 36   Polygram 68t   Popperfoto 30; 31   Mark Power 98l   Private Stock Records 85   David Redfern 55; 74r Peter Cronin   Rex Features 57r; 58; 59b   RCA 66; 67; 93   The Rickster 107b   Derek Ridgers 87; 92t; 83 (inset)   Douglas Robertson 96   Sheila Rock 35   Penny Ryder Publicity/Vidal Sassoon 53tl, ml, b; 73   Jon Savage 52m   Kate Simon 63   Penny Smith 98r   Neil Spencer 50m   Sporting Pictures (UK) Ltd 110/111   Kark Stoecker 65   Graeme Montgomery/Sunday Times 110m   Syndication International 61   The Tate Gallery, London 17   Dave Taylor 27   Topham 80bl   Virginia Turbett 92b   United Artists 11t   Virgin 101b   Warner Bros 102b   Alfred Wertheimer 23   Nick White 90   Russell Young 100b   Antenna (photo Mike Owen)/EMI Records (photo Paul Rider) cover

Bibliography

Barnes, Richard, *Mods!*, 1979
Bernard, Barbara, *Fashion in the Sixties*, 1978
Best, Pete and Patrick Doncaster, *Beatle! The Pete Best Story*, 1985
Billy Boy, *Barbie*, 1987
Bockris, Victor and Gerald Malenga, *Up-Tight*, 1983
Bones, Jah, *One Love*, 1985
Bowie, Angie, *Free Spirit*, 1981
Burchill, Julie, *Girls on Film*, 1986
Carmichael, Stokely, *Stokely Speaks*, 1971
Carr, Roy, Brian Case and Fred Dellar, *The Hip*, 1986
Cohen, Stanley, *Folk Devils and Moral Panics*, 1972
Cohn, Nik, *Awopbobaloobop! Alopbamboom!* 1969
Cohn, Nik, *Today There Are No Gentlemen*, 1971
Coleridge, Nicholas, *The Fashion Conspiracy*, 1988
Corson, Richard, *Fashions In Hair*, 1980
Dalton, David, *The Mutant King*, 1974
Dalton, David and Ron Cayen, *James Dean: American Icon*, 1984
Edelstein, Andrew J., *The Pop Sixties*, 1985
Everett, Peter, *You'll Never Be 16 Again*, 1986
Goldman, Albert, *Elvis*, 1979
Grogan, Emmett, *Ringolevio*, 1972
Hebdige, Dick, *Subculture*, 1979
Hopkins, Jerry, Jim Marshall, and Baron Welman, *Festival!* 1970
Hunter, Allan, *Tony Curtis*, 1985
Hunter, Ian, *Diary of a Rock'n'Roll Star*, 1974
Jones, Mablen, *Getting It On*, 1987
Kelley, Kitty, *His Way*, 1986
Knight, Nick, *Skinhead*, 1982
Mercer, Kobena, *Black Hair/Style Politics*, 1987
Lewis, Peter, *The Fifties*, 1978
Mailer, Norman *Advertisements For Myself*, 1961
Macpherson, Don and Louise Brody, *Leading Ladies*, 1986
Malcolm X, *The Autobiography of Malcolm X*, 1965
Melly, George, *Revolt into Style*, 1972
Mungham, Geoff (ed.) and Geoff Pearson, *Working Class Youth Culture*, 1976
Norman, Philip, *Shout!*, 1981
Peellaert, Guy, and Nik Cohn, *Rock Dreams*, 1973
Polhemus, Ted and Lynn Procter, *Pop Styles*, 1984
Stallings, Penny, *Rock'n'Roll Confidential*, 1984
Steele-Perkins, Chris, and Richard Smith, *The Teds*, 1987
Stern, Jane and Michael, *Elvis World*, 1987
Stuart, Johnny, *Rockers*, 1987
Toop, David, *The Rap Attack*, 1984
Twiggy, *Twiggy*, 1975
Weisbord, Robert G., *Ebony Kinship – Africa, Africans and the Afro American*, 1973
Wilson, Mary, *Dreamgirl*, 1986
Wolfe, Tom, *Radical Chic and Mau-Mauing the Flak Catchers*, 1971
Wolfe, Tom, *Mauve Gloves and Madmen, Clutter and Vine*, 1976
Wolfe, Tom, *In Our Time*, 1980
Wroblewski, Chris, and Nelly Gommez-Vaez, *City Indians*, 1984
York, Peter, *Modern Times*, 1984
York, Peter, *Style Wars*, 1980
Zanetta, Tony and Henry Edwards, *Stardust*, 1986

Magazines and Journals

Elegant Hair; The Face, The Hairdressers' Journal, i-D, Life; Newsweek; New Musical Express; Rolling Stone; Time.